-5-05

Benjamin P. Bowser
Shiraz I. Mishra
Cathy J. Reback
George F. Lemp
Editors

Preventing AIDS
Community-Science
Collaborations

Pre-publication
REVIEWS,
COMMENTARIES,
EVALUATIONS . . .

"**F**or everyone interested in HIV prevention, or in the growing discourse concerning practice-research collaboration in the behavioral sciences, *Preventing AIDS: Community-Science Collaborations* is among the most important books to emerge this year. The book begins with a uniquely readable, thoughtful, and historically grounded discussion of observational research to describe how the scientific enterprise is often unhinged from community-based organizations and the populations they serve, and to forcefully explain the need for collaboration. The second chapter details how two funding agencies worked to draw both community-based organizations and researchers into equal part-nerships that would better serve the goals of improving prevention strategies for difficult-to-reach populations. The remaining chapters report case studies of individual community-science collaborations concerned with HIV prevention among injection drug users, sex workers, migrant farmworkers, prison inmates, street youths, and transgender persons. 'What needs to happen is obvious,' the authors conclude. 'The community needs to become more central to research efforts' and '[r]esearchers need to use their knowledge to rigorously and sensitively evaluate program efforts.' By example, and through the voices of community service providers, researchers, and funders, this book tells us how."

Joseph Guydish, PhD
Adjunct Professor of Medicine
and Health Policy Studies,
University of California, San Francisco

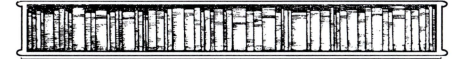

More pre-publication
REVIEWS, COMMENTARIES, EVALUATIONS . . .

"**A**t National Development and Research Institutes, we work with service providers, youths, and drug users around health issues, HIV/AIDS, hepatitis C, drug treatment, and many other issues. We are constantly seeking ways to build more effective collaborations. The case studies and ideas in *Preventing AIDS: Community-Science Collaborations* will help us do a better job. For this, I want to thank the editors very deeply."

Samuel R. Friedman, PhD
Senior Research Fellow,
Institute for AIDS Research;
Director, Social Theory Core,
Center for Drug Use and HIV Research,
National Development
and Research Institutes,
New York City

The Haworth Press®
New York • London • Oxford

Preventing AIDS
Community-Science
Collaborations

Haworth Psychosocial Issues of HIV/AIDS
R. Dennis Shelby, PhD
Senior Editor

Preventing AIDS
Community-Science Collaborations

Benjamin P. Bowser
Shiraz I. Mishra
Cathy J. Reback
George F. Lemp
Editors

The Haworth Press®
New York • London • Oxford

PUBLISHER'S NOTE
Identities and circumstances of individuals discussed in this book have been changed to protect confidentiality.

The Haworth Press, Inc., 10 Alice Street, Binghamton, NY 13904-1580.

Cover design by Jennifer M. Gaska.

Library of Congress Cataloging-in-Publication Data

Preventing AIDS : community-science collaborations / Benjamin P. Bowser . . . [et al.], editors.
    p. cm.
    ISBN 0-7890-1234-0 (Hard : alk. paper) — ISBN 0-7890-1247-2 (Soft : alk. paper)
    1. AIDS (Disease)—Prevention. 2. AIDS (Disease)—Prevention—Research—California.
3. Public health—Research—Methodology. I. Bowser, Benjamin P.

RA643.8.P74 2004
362.196'9792—dc22
                                                        2003026556

CONTENTS

ABOUT THE EDITORS

Benjamin P. Bowser, PhD, is Professor of Sociology and Social Services and Director of the Urban Institute at California State University, Hayward. He has published on issues of race and racism for over twenty years and is co-editor of the now classic *Impacts of Racism on White Americans* and *Against the Odds: Scholars Who Challenged Racism in the Twentieth Century.* He also does extensive community-based research on HIV/AIDS prevention with grants from the U.S. Centers for Disease Control, The Robert Wood Johnson Foundation, The University of California, and The National Institute on Drug Abuse. He was guest editor of "The Social Dimensions of the AIDS Epidemic: A Sociology of the AIDS Epidemic" for the *International Journal of Sociology and Social Policy.*

Shiraz I. Mishra, MD, PhD, is Association Professor of Epidemiology and Preventive Medicine and Deputy Director at the Office of Policy and Planning's Maryland Statewide Health Network at the University of Maryland at Baltimore School of Medicine. He is co-editor of *AIDS Crossing Borders: The Spread of HIV Among Migrant Latinos* and has numerous peer-reviewed publications. Dr. Mishra's research has made important contributions toward understanding health disparities, especially chronic diseases such as HIV/AIDS, as experienced by ethnic/racial minorities in the United States and internationally.

Cathy J. Reback, PhD, is Director of the Prevention Division at the Van Ness Recovery House and a principal investigator at Friends Research Institute, Inc. Dr. Reback has been a principal investigator or co-principal investigator on projects funded by NIDA, CSAT, UARP, and the City of Los Angeles. She has also served as director of service projects funded by the County of Los Angeles, Office of AIDS Programs and Policy, and the City of West Hollywood.

George F. Lemp, DRPH, MPH, has been director of the University-wide AIDS Research Program at the University of California, Office of the President, since 1995. Prior to this position, Dr. Lemp served for nine years as chief of the AIDS Epidemiology and Surveillance Branch at the San Francisco Department of Public Health. He has also been affiliated with the National Institute of Health. Dr. Lemp has been author or co-author of nearly fifty published articles in a variety of journals covering topics on HIV/AIDS or other diseases.

CONTRIBUTORS

Bart K. Aoki, PhD, is a clinical psychologist who has worked in mental health, substance abuse, and HIV/AIDS service settings and has conducted community-based evaluation research with diverse ethnic/racial communities. Currently, he is associate director and co-ordinator, Social-Behavioral and Health Sciences Research at the Universitywide AIDS Research Program, University of California, Office of the President.

Dante Brimer was a core staff interviewer and outreach worker on the UFO field site team. He was a founding member of The Horribles, a San Francisco suit- and tie-clad punk posse, still infamous among Haight-Ashbury street youths. Also known as the Les Paul-slinging-guitar-playing heartthrob of the rock band "Mack Truck," Dante played to packed audiences all over town, and made *All Right!!!* the band's first CD on Wear It Low Records. Known to his friends as El Dante, his fans as Dante Mack, and to his family as Benjamin Brimer III, he stole hearts and won laughs everywhere he went. A fine human being, a brilliant problem solver, and a young man with an intellect and intuition as big as his heart, Dante was a pure joy. We miss him more than words can say.

Ross F. Conner, PhD, is the director of the Center for Community Health Research, University of California, Irvine, and an associate professor, Department of Planning, Policy, and Design in the School of Social Ecology at UCI. He received his PhD and MA from Northwestern University (social psychology/evaluation) and his BA from Johns Hopkins University. His most recent book is *AIDS: Science and Society* (with H. Fan and L. Villarreal); he has cowritten or co-edited eight other books, as well as numerous papers and reports. His research focuses on community health promotion/disease prevention programs. Ross is the past president of the American Evaluation Association. He also works with various foundations, government agencies, and organizations on evaluation and community health issues.

Carla Dillard-Smith, MPA, is deputy and research director of the California Prostitute Education Program (CAL-PEP). Besides providing fiscal and program oversight, she provides coordination and programmatic direction to various CAL-PEP ethnographic research projects in support of AIDS care, treatment, and prevention education to high-risk populations in the San Francisco East Bay and city.

Heather Edney-Meschery served as the executive director of the Santa Cruz County Needle Exchange Program for thirteen years. In addition to serving as coinvestigator on countless research projects, Ms. Edney-Meschery also developed and implemented cutting-edge prevention programs that have been replicated nationwide ranging from hepatitis C and overdose prevention to a countywide sharps disposal program. She is also the managing editor of *Junkphood,* a low-cost magazine written by and for the injection-drug-using community with worldwide distribution.

Bonnie Faigeles was senior statistician at UCSF Center for AIDS Prevention Studies (CAPS). She has participated in several community-based research collaborations apart from her work with Centerforce. Currently, Ms. Faigeles is a student at the UCSF School of Nursing.

Olga Grinstead, PhD, MPH, is an adjunct associate professor at UCSF School of Medicine and Center for AIDS Prevention Studies (CAPS). Her research involves the development, implementation, and evaluation of HIV prevention programs in collaboration with community service providers. As director of CAPS' Technology and Information Exchange Core, she also promotes and facilitates community collaborative research and the development of best practices for HIV prevention and evaluation of community-based HIV prevention programs. Dr. Grinstead is also a licensed clinical psychologist.

Lisa M. Krieger is an award-winning journalist in the San Francisco Bay area, where for seventeen years she has covered medical news for *The San Francisco Examiner* and the *San Jose Mercury News.* A graduate of Duke University, she was contributing editor to *Incredible Voyage: Exploring The Human Body* by National Geographic Press. She lives in Palo Alto, California, with her daughter.

Gloria Lockett is founder and executive director of the California Prostitute Education Program (CAL-PEP), which is the largest street outreach and direct service HIV/AIDS prevention organization in the San Francisco East Bay. CAL-PEP has pioneered a number of street outreach techniques to reach hard-to-access HIV/AIDS risk groups.

Services include safer-sex and needle-use workshops for sex workers, IV, and other drug users, juveniles, and prisoners. CAL-PEP also runs a risk-reduction day-treatment center for women who abuse drugs.

Rachel McLean, BS. In memory of the clients and colleagues that she has lost to overdose, Ms. McLean founded the Drug Overdose Prevention and Education (DOPE) Project. The DOPE Project trains injection drug users, treatment providers, and criminal justice personnel in overdose recognition, response, and prevention, and advocates for structural change to reduce overdose deaths in San Francisco. DOPE is currently collaborating with the Department of Public Health to implement a model naloxone distribution program.

Andrew Moss, PhD, is a professor of epidemiology and biostatistics and professor of medicine at UCSF, and was principal investigator of the UFO study of young injectors 1997-2002. He has been working in the epidemiology of AIDS and related fields since 1982.

Roger K. Myrick, PhD, is the senior prevention evaluation scientist at the Universitywide AIDS Research Program, Office of the President, University of California. In this capacity, Dr. Myrick coordinates the collaborative prevention evaluation program and serves as a research liaison to the California State Office of AIDS. Dr. Myrick's research interests include community collaborative research and prevention evaluation for gay men.

Lisa Netherland is manager for HIV Prevention Services for the San Mateo County Health Services Agency in California. She is the co-chair of the HIV Prevention Planning Group of San Mateo County and is the project director for the Door to Treatment project, a substance abuse treatment intervention to reduce HIV risk among chronic drug users. She has extensive experience in women's health including work as a trainer, educator, and administrator in the areas of domestic violence, lesbian health, chemical dependency, incarceration, and sexually transmitted diseases. She is a graduate of the University of Illinois, Urbana-Champaign.

Kristen Ochoa is a medical student at the University of Southern California, Keck School of Medicine. Prior to attending medical school, Kristen worked for twelve years in the field of HIV and substance use at the San Francisco AIDS Foundation, the Haight-Ashbury Free Medical Clinic, and UCSF's Department of Epidemiology and Biostatistics. She has presented and published widely on needle exchange, HIV, hepatitis, heroin overdose, and injection drug use among youths. She is currently researching the impact of soft tissue infections on needle exchangers in Skid Row, Los Angeles.

Geraldine Oliva, MD, MPH, is an adjunct associate professor of family and community medicine, a member of the Institute for Health Policy Studies at the University of California at San Francisco, and the director of the Family Health Outcomes Project (FHOP). Dr. Oliva is a board-certified pediatrician with a broad background as a clinician, public health administrator, and researcher. Before creating FHOP in 1992, she directed the development and operation of the Adolescent Medicine Program at Children's Hospital in Oakland, California, served as medical director of the San Francisco/Alameda Planned Parenthood affiliate, and served as family health director and then deputy director for community health at the San Francisco Department of Pubic Health.

Jennifer Rienks, MS, PhD(c), is an analyst with the Family Health Outcomes Project in the Department of Family and Community Medicine at the University of California, San Francisco. Ms. Rienks received her training in social psychology and is currently working to complete her PhD. Ms. Rienks' research interests include using social psychological theories to develop and test interventions designed to encourage individual health-related behavior change and collective action to change health policies and social norms in groups experiencing health disparities. Currently, Ms. Rienks is working on evaluating a project to reduce disparities in infant mortality. She has also worked on projects addressing cancer and diabetes disparities in the African-American community, and evaluated a cancer patient navigator program.

Fernando Sanudo is the cofounder of the Vista Community Clinic Health Promotion Center. Initiated in 1987, the Health Promotion Center houses over forty grant-funded programs and employs seventy full- and part-time staff. In the past fifteen years, he has researched, designed, implemented, and evaluated a myriad of community-health programs focused on multicultural populations. Because of his expertise in program design and evaluation, Mr. Sanudo has been invited to consult and/or review proposals for the following organizations: The California Endowment, The San Diego Foundation, County of San Diego Office of AIDS, University of California Irvine, Tri-City Medical Center, Universitywide AIDS Research Program, and the Centers for Disease Control. He has a bachelor's degree in biology from the University of California, San Diego, and a master's degree in public health (MPH) with a concentration in health promotion from San Diego State University.

Paul Simon, MD, MPH, is Director, Health Assessment and Epidemiology, Los Angeles County Department of Health Services and an adjunct associated professor, Department of Epidemiology, UCLA School of Public Health. His primary research interests are in public health surveillance and population health tracking.

Steve Truax, PhD, is a research psychologist who works in basic and applied research in university and applied settings in mental and general health. Currently, he is the chief of the HIV Prevention Research and Evaluation Section at the California Department of Health, Office of AIDS.

Barry Zack, MPH, is the executive director of Centerforce, a community-based agency working with incarcerated populations and their families. Since 1986, he has been working with inmates on health-related issues (HIV, hepatitis, and other STIs), and currently leads agency efforts with prisoner, transitional, and child/family programs. Mr. Zack has been involved in community-based research since 1989; approximately 30 percent of Centerforce's efforts are research related, providing the agency with ongoing input to increase program/intervention effectiveness.

Preface

In Chapter 2, The University of California, University-wide AIDS Research Program (UARP) calls for proposals to fund CREPC projects. The UARP program directors tell why and how they devised such a unique funding opportunity. In a rare inside view of the funders, we learn the politics and the administrative twists and turns that were necessary to offer such funding. In the next section of this book are the core case studies illustrating projects that varied in the extent to which they were able to achieve the CREPC balance between research and community.

The projects in Chapters 3 through 5 show the power and advantage of collaborative research in which the researcher and community-based partners were able to cooperatively plan and execute AIDS prevention projects. In Chapter 3 Gloria Lockett and Carla Dillard-Smith at Oakland's CAL-PEP discuss how they worked with Benjamin Bowser at California State University, Hayward, to assess their work. Here, the focus was not only on evaluating CAL-PEP's program effectiveness. The staff had long-held ideas and insights on why their clients were in the streets and why they were clients in the first place. Besides their program, they wanted their ideas explored in precisely the area that most AIDS prevention research has missed—a comprehensive study of why high-risk people are at high risk in the first place. In Chapter 4, Fernando Sanudo and a team at Vista Community Clinic in Vista, California, worked with Shiraz Mishra at the University of California, Irvine. This is a community-based study that uses near classical experimental methods done in isolated migrant farmworker camps across Southern California. They show the power of combining qualitative with quantitative techniques.

In Chapter 5, Barry Zack of the Marin AIDS Project worked with Olga Grinstead of the University of California, San Francisco. Prison environments are one of the most difficult to work in because the rules regarding access to prisoners can change at a moment's notice. This team shows how they were able to use the extraordinary knowledge and access of the Marin AIDS Project team to craft a rigorous project despite multiple changes in access to prisoners. In Chapter 6, Cathy Reback and a team at the Van Ness Recovery House worked with Paul Simon of the Los Angeles County Department of Health. This may be one of the few collaborative studies to look at one of the most hard-to-access of all populations, transgendered persons. In Chapter 7, Lisa Netherland and a team at Golden Gate Planned Parenthood joined with Gerry Oliva at The University of California, San Francisco. The CREPC collaborative research illustrated by this study was the third in a series of linked studies. This is a very important chapter because it shows, in the second of the three studies, what happens if the research is not done collaboratively. You will notice that the third and collaborative part of the study had fewer surprises and generated better data.

In Chapter 8, Kristen Ochoa and a community research team joined efforts with Andrew Moss, both with San Francisco General Hospital. They did a prevention study of street youths in San Francisco's Haight and Mission Districts. This is the most sensitive record of the inner tensions and conflicts between the service providers' service role and the requirements to conduct research. As in the prior studies, we see the advantages and problems inherent in having the service provider fully responsible for the research. In the first part of Chapter 9, Benjamin Bowser and Lisa Krieger distill the research lessons learned from conducting community researcher equal partner collaborations (CREPC). In the second part of Chapter 9, the community service lessons learned are discussed. Then, in Chapter 10, the importance of CREPC is discussed along with what are the next steps in further developing CREPC.

Chapter 1

Introduction to Community-Science Collaboration: Equal Partners in Investigation

Benjamin P. Bowser
Shiraz I. Mishra

COLLABORATION

Collaborations between community-based service providers and university-based researchers are rare. If attempted, they are difficult to sustain. But the benefits of such collaborations can result in both richer science and improved delivery of urgent services to troubled populations.

This book describes advancement in the way that social and behavioral sciences are conducted. It shows how to broaden the range of basic research that can be done in applied settings and mixes quantitative and qualitative methods. Equally significant, it shows how important principles of collaboration can be applied to the work of community-based organizations in using research to improve their services, work more effectively with their clients, and build technical capacity (Israel et al., 1998).

This book is for anyone interested in using the art of collaboration to bring scientific solutions to human problems. Innovations in conducting research and creating interventions to solve social issues seldom make the science section of *The New York Times*. Yet they profoundly affect how we think about one another and ourselves and influence the ways that business is conducted and social services are provided. The specific mission of this book is to take a close look, from multiple perspectives, at how a collaboration has substantially contributed to reductions of epidemic rates of HIV infections and

1

AIDS in the United States (Becker and Joseph, 1988; Gibson, McCusker, and Chesney, 1998; Normand, Vlahov, and Moses, 1995; Sloboda, 1998).

The term "collaborative research" has become increasingly popular in recent years as people and organizations, once strangers to one another, have recognized the benefits of working together to promote public health. This book focuses on a specific form of collaborative research between university-based researchers and community-based organizations dedicated to HIV/AIDS prevention. However, the collaborative technique we describe is not limited to AIDS prevention work. It can be applied to problem solving in a host of areas.

Central to a successful collaboration is the premise that both groups work as equal partners in investigation, described as "community-researcher equal partner collaboration" (CREPC). The principles of such collaborations have already been outlined. Before portraying various collaborative efforts, we will look at a short history of the way social and behavioral scientists and community-based practitioners usually go about their work. Collaboration, in contrast, offers advancement of both research and community service practices.

Conventional Approaches

What Researchers Do

A broad spectrum of techniques is used to conduct social and behavioral research. These range from complex mathematical models based upon large data sets to general observations of a single social setting—a bar, restaurant, or street corner.

Most of the work done in HIV/AIDS prevention falls in the middle, using neither large-scale sampling nor a single observation. Although it does not come out of a strong tradition of formal theory, it is not without theory. A particular challenge in HIV/AIDS prevention is that it is impossible to identify and interview everyone who is at risk or who engages in risky behaviors. It is impossible not simply because of the numbers and variety of people but because sexual behavior and drug use are private and hidden behaviors; they are further hidden when they are stigmatized or considered deviant. This is why much prevention research is done in agencies, organizations, and residential communities.

In HIV/AIDS and all other forms of human social research, sampling strategies are the most well-known and preferred quantitative approach to research since World War II (Hammersley, 1992). Scientists have relied on this strategy as the best way to derive evidence of "representative" behavior, attitudes, and opinions (Bebbie, 1990). In other words, an interview of everyone in a community would not reveal any more information than what is obtained using a carefully crafted, smaller, and more cost efficient random sample. In contrast, observational strategies such as ethnography, focus groups, and using key informants are qualitative research strategies that fell out of favor after World War II. Used on the margins of the disciplines for decades, they are now experiencing renewed interest (Guba, 1990).

Trained investigators, who by habit and tradition do not require people outside of the research team to be involved in the research process, generally plan sampling procedures and define the research questions. Bias and not following procedure are very real concerns that compromise the integrity of analysis. In projects in which it is necessary to interview respondents one-on-one in the community, "field sites" are often set up to develop a presence in the community. People and organizations in these communities are sought out to provide access and a site. When this data-oriented quantitative technique was first employed in the 1920s, residents were very cooperative and generally respectful of the people and agencies that sponsored the research (Converse, 1987). But problems were apparent right from the beginning (Hyman and Singer, 1991). What if the distribution of households in the community did not also approximate the distribution of population in that community? In central city communities with large numbers of racial and ethnic groups, only the more affluent, the very old, and the very young were accessed through random household surveys. There was then, as now, no way to completely enumerate the population in these communities in order to select a random sample. Also, most residents in these more complex city communities did not trust outsiders and only saw interviews as nuisances.

Today, the problem of accessing people cuts across social and ethnic strata. For example, there are people with multiple homes, no homes, and most are rarely at home. It is not unusual to have post office boxes as home addresses, security guards who screen visitors in the lobby, and coded intercom systems that prevent direct access to building residents. In addition, answering machines, fax and data lines, and message centers further frustrate access by telephone. Furthermore, busy people on the run are not going to give interviews from their cell phones. What if, in addition to all these modern barriers to access, the very people you must study see researchers in the same way as they see junk mail, unsolicited advertisers, or the police? They will work hard to avoid contact with such people. Because of the increasing difficulty of getting systematic data, there has been a revival of interest in qualitative research methods (Guba, 1990) that rely on observational techniques (Agar, 1986; Denzin and Lincoln, 1998), and there is an evolving effort to pragmatically combine quantitative and qualitative research designs (Tashakkori and Teddie, 1998).

With more barriers to access each year, community-based samples are increasingly difficult to get and very expensive to conduct. Researchers outside of HIV/AIDS prevention projects avoid having to collect community samples. But what if one's research requires access to very difficult-to-reach subpopulations in specific communities? How do you reach people who are not only inaccessible through traditional means, but who also have reasons to avoid being interviewed? Injection drug users, and sex workers, for example, are not likely to admit to these behaviors.

Qualitative, not quantitative, techniques are better suited for gaining information about hard-to-access populations, such as information about social settings, and understanding behaviors (Agar, 1986; Lofland and Lofland, 1995). But reaching hard-to-access populations, even when using qualitative techniques, now requires working with the people and organizations that routinely work with them (Johnson, 1990). In HIV and AIDS prevention, these are agencies that the at-risk population trusts because they offer information and services. These qualitative methods must be used to gain knowledge and insight into a population and its surrounding environment before more structured quantitative methods can be employed (Lambert, Ashery, and Needle, 1995).

No tradition of collaboration exists to bring to these new working relationships. Furthermore, not all researchers are convinced of the importance of collaboration, beyond gaining access to a research site and difficult-to-reach populations.

What Community-Based HIV/AIDS Agencies Do

Community service organizations in the United States usually begin as volunteer groups who see a social need and feel compelled to respond (Bowser, 1998; Cox, 1994; Hoffman, 1989). The work and advocacy of each new movement often forces governments to respond with funding to address the problem by expanding services. But the amount of money that is provided is invariably a fraction of what is needed. The HIV/AIDS prevention movement is a case in point. The original AIDS prevention organizations started as volunteer groups with the mission to arrest the AIDS epidemic in their specific communities and among specific risk-taking groups. Their volunteers often come from the at-risk groups or from people who worked closely with them prior to the epidemic (Van Vugt, 1994). The service area is generally very specific as is the service population. This is because the effectiveness of a community-specific service is highly dependent upon having intimate knowledge, access to, and the trust of the HIV risk subcommunity. This knowledge, access, and trust are not necessarily interchangeable from neighborhood to neighborhood. In addition, there are ethnic, lifestyle, racial, and social class boundaries that are not easily crossed (Bowser, 1994).

Once government funding becomes available, larger and already established community-based agencies step in. Although established to address prior crises, they begin AIDS prevention services by hiring prevention activists and others concerned with stopping the AIDS epidemic. Once organized, HIV/AIDS prevention requires outreach to the community's high-risk groups. Outreach workers, who are poorly paid and work in whole communities, are the front line. Their services are absolutely dependent upon successful and continuous access to the high-risk group whether outreach works from a fixed site, by walking the streets, or by mobile van. In effect, the service has to be offered where the at-risk group is; prevention agencies cannot wait for high-risk individuals to come to them.

Stigma is attached to people who work with those with HIV and AIDS (Davis, 1995) so association with an AIDS service organization is not a socially neutral event. As a result, outreach workers have to develop social ties and relationships one at a time. Often, they have to provide other services—services they are not funded to provide—to avoid stigmatizing clients and to develop an identity broader than just

AIDS services. Many drug users are engaged in illegal activities, such as purchasing and selling illegal drugs, possessing needles and syringes without a prescription, and committing crime to support their drug habit. So drug users are "underground," often have warrants for their arrest, and are very busy maintaining their drug habit and the social relationships that support their habit. Finally, the highest risk people are more often people living in poverty. Their lives are unpredictable, they have to survive day to day, they do not necessarily have jobs, and they are often in crisis. The bottom line is that services must go where the clients are and be available when they are open to receive them.

Clearly, accessing people in bathhouses, on street corners, in crack houses, in homeless camps, and in single occupancy hotels is not traditional work. Not everyone can do it. At minimum, outreach requires street smarts, high verbal skills and humor, the capacity to accept people for who they are and in whatever condition they are in, and not being easily intimidated. One has to know when to stand one's ground and when not to. This is a different world from that of people who work in offices and who live in mainstream society. Researchers cannot simply walk into this world and start asking questions. Ironically, people who live in the underground are often very familiar with what past researchers have done. They remember prior study findings that clearly show no knowledge or insight into their lives and communities. Needless to say, research and researchers are not highly regarded, and are looked upon by those in need, as well as those who provide the services, with suspicion and avoidance.

At the same time, most service providers have no way to directly demonstrate that they are effective and are making a positive difference in their clients' lives. The ability to be where high-risk people are, to really talk with them, and to empathize with their plight is not enough in itself to change HIV risk behaviors. A real service—something that works—must be provided. A service that may have worked in one community may not work as well in some other community (Van Vugt, 1994). Even in the same community, a service that works at one time may not work at some other time in the same community. This is because high-risk populations can change rapidly with the introduction of new drugs as happened with crack cocaine in the mid-1980s. Also, new subgroups can become HIV infected and require a different approach to outreach. So the questions of relative effectiveness and impact must be addressed, and not simply to appease funders. More important, it is necessary to constantly review and revise outreach and treatment strategies to keep them effective. Therefore, community-based organizations, in an effort to maximize their services and impact, must work with organizations with the skills required to not only evaluate services, but to understand changing community needs.

Compromise and Cooperation

The preferred way to get rigorous representative data on community populations simply does not work as intended. Direct random samples are often out of the question because of the difficulty in determining population parameters. Therefore, it is necessary to work through people who have access to hard-to-reach populations; without that, the best one can do is get "convenience" or "snowball" samples (Watters, 1993). Interviewing hard-to-access populations poses a challenge to interviewers as well. Not all well-trained interviewers are prepared to conduct interviews on the streets, in their cars, in alleys, in crack houses, or wherever respondents are. To reach hard-to-access, at-risk groups, interviewers must carry themselves well in the underground, deal with challenges to their presence, carry subject payment, and conduct interviews in inconvenient and potentially dangerous locations. If they show fear, disgust, impatience, or shock, they can influence and compromise their interviews. Research in such settings often requires that the service agency use their outreach staff to recruit clients for interviews. Potential respondents need to be approached, convinced to participate, and assured of the interview's value. They must trust that the interview is confidential and supported by the service agency and staff. Then the interviewer must be introduced and spoken for by the service staff. Recruiters or any other intermediates between the interviewer and respondent add yet another challenge to the research, because they can influence the research outcomes with biased selection, or bias the client-respondent toward the interview or interviewer.

Instead of having complete control over the interview and research, research investigators find with each twist and turn in the field that they are dependent upon their community partner. This further challenges the ideal research model. The new reality is that the researcher has access because of the service agency's sponsorship. This is not a casual event. The service providers must convince their clients to be interviewed, and to offer accurate and truthful information when interviewed. The service agency and staff put their reputations and, more often, fragile relationships with clients on the line to give the researchers and interviewers temporary access to them. It may have taken the service provider years to establish trust and a working relationship with its clients. Service agencies, therefore, want some assurance that the interviewers and researchers are sensitive to the social environment, will respect and not abuse the agency's extension of trust, and recognize that after the research is complete and they have gone, the agency must still continue its work and relationships with clients.

Researchers who do not understand or accept the complexity of the communities they want to work in attempt to stay in control of all aspects of the project. They do not work cooperatively with their community host. A common mistake among researchers is to think that they can simply pay the service provider for access to their clients. Such researchers then insist upon supervising interviewers, recruiters, and anyone else on site to ensure a high-quality interview. They do not realize that the quality of both the recruitment and interviews is critically dependent upon the morale and buy in of clients, recruiters, and interviewers, regardless of "who is in control." The interviews do not get done well simply because one pays staff. The quality and accuracy of what is gained can be seriously compromised if the field team and agency staff does not have a personal stake and sense of involvement in the research. Some university and public health departments will attempt to create their own community-based agencies by expanding their clinic outreach to get around the problem of collaboration. In doing so, they may avoid the need to work with a partner, but still face the challenge of getting hard-to-access populations in sufficient numbers, something an independent partner with considerable outreach experience can do very well (Gubrium and Silverman, 1989).

From the point of view of community-based organizations, why do they need researchers to evaluate their work? After all, they have access to high-risk populations and know the communities they operate in. They know the people who have benefited from their services and can tell you about them. This should be sufficient evidence that they have made a difference, and each year the list of successes grows. Furthermore, they know why their work has succeeded and made a difference, and can list the barriers they have overcome to be effective. Agencies are capable of summarizing their successes. They can also list where their services are deficient and what they need to do to improve them, if provided the resources to do so. AIDS community-based service organizations are also aware that in other professions, self-study and assessment are acceptable. So why do they need outsiders coming in to research what they already know? They may perceive that assessment research is a waste of time and money, and may suspect that the findings will be used against them. The fact that funders are starting to link independent assessment with continued funding is viewed as a barrier to their work. They often believe that money spent on research could be better used to expand services.

An alternative view exists among other community-based agencies. Some agencies are very much aware of the limits of their work, have a lot of unanswered questions about their clientele and communities, and see value in ensuring that they are operating as effectively as possible. They also realize that they need to be able to generate systematic data and reports on their client population in order to better compete for expanded funding and the development of new programs. But limits on funding and staffing prevent them from creating such assessments on their own. These agencies are receptive to working with outsiders to do two things: improve their internal capacity to do research and self-assessments, and provide independent assessments of their work. An added benefit might be getting their own questions answered about their clientele and communities. They know that the match between themselves and the researcher is very important. Within an agency, those who view research with suspicion and those who see it as a potential benefit might struggle over which view dominates. Increasingly, the proactive view is winning the day—especially if evaluation can increase the agency's capacity to do research, compete for funding, upgrade computers, and improve staff skills.

CREPC

What is community-researcher equal partner collaboration (CREPC) and why is it an important innovation? CREPC brings people from two very different and conflicting communities together to work for a common goal. Community agencies and the social and behavioral sciences consist of worlds unto themselves. Most psychologists and sociologists do not work with people in residential communities as an intrinsic part of their careers. The essence of pure social and behavioral sciences is exploration of any topic based upon free inquiry unencumbered by the need for applications (Carey, 1989). But this is a far cry from the reality of the field (Gubrium and Silverman, 1989). The research "community" is a privileged world of people with advanced degrees, who are relatively affluent, and highly selective of what they do. The research community is based in universities and colleges, and increasingly in businesses, government agencies, and research institutes (Converse, 1987). Of course, some people bridge the residential community and the research world and are interested in applying their training and the sciences to improving society; but their worldview does not dominate.

The second community that is a part of CREPC is social service providers—it too is large, diverse, and has its own specializations, missions, and purposes. Social service communities are not strangers to research. More often, when they serve as extensions of university departments and government agencies, they too engage in research. They provide a setting and context to apply science to social problems. However, most social service providers are not government agencies or parts of universities. They are residential, community-based organizations created to respond to some social problem within their community such as alcohol abuse, child welfare, housing, health, education, drug treatment, and, more recently, HIV/AIDS prevention (Van Vugt, 1994). They are often founded by community leaders and are staffed by people who have experienced the problem firsthand. They have boards of directors made up of residents of their service community. They have missions that express their racial, ethnic, religious, lifestyle, and social class backgrounds. These are not the same communities that most scientists are from or live in. Furthermore, these communities have the most extensive social problems, are less privileged, and more often segregated from mainstream society. Residentially based agencies in such underprivileged communities are generally referred to as "community-based organizations" (CBOs). Their ongoing and enduring commitment to serve people in need makes them important.

Central Problem Addressed

The central problem addressed by this book is twofold. First, few residential community-based organizations use existing scientific knowledge to improve and advance their services, although there are exceptions (Lamb, Greenlick, and McCarty, 1989). Like their clients, they tend to be suspicious of science and scientists. They do not want to have their clients and communities exploited and left with nothing to show for participation in studies. They do not want to be misunderstood and then described negatively in published studies. Second, few scientists, who wish to address urgent social problems, have the trust of the people with the problems, nor do they have ways to reach them. The interested scientists cannot bring their expertise and methods to solve social problems without access to the people and communities where the problems are. Furthermore, the scientific method requires control over data, precision, impartiality, and independence from participants and nonscience collaborators. A result is a gap between the immediate interests of residentially based community organizations and the methods of scientific inquiry. This gap compromises progress in effectively addressing social problems, whether the problem is alcohol and drug addiction, poor education, crime prevention, or preventing the spread of HIV/AIDS.

Community-researcher equal partner collaborations (CREPC) successfully address this impasse between communities and scientists (Israel et al., 1998). But it requires the following:

1. Both parties must wish to address a common problem and agree on a solution. In this book, the common goal was to slow down, perhaps prevent, the spread of HIV/AIDS among hard-to-reach, high-risk groups.
2. Both parties must understand that neither party can achieve the goal without the other.
3. The CBO director and the researcher(s) must be equal partners in authority as coinvestigators.
4. Each party must be fully involved in the planning, design, and execution of the project, as well as interpretation of results.
5. A mutual agreement must be reached about the end product such as publications, reports, training manuals, staff enhancement, and training as well as agreement about who keeps equip-

ment (computers, software, and office furniture) after the project is completed.

6. Mutual trust must be achieved through regular meetings to address problems, a willingness to learn the concerns and limits of the other party, and flexibility in problem solving.

7. Researchers must understand that community collaborators have valid hypotheses, theories, and insights to contribute to the research, based upon their experience with their client population.

Community-research teams that work within these principles will work well together. The researcher must work with the CBO to develop a methodology that is appropriate for their organization, clients, and community, involving the CBO director and staff in the planning process. The CBO must take partial ownership of the project. The researchers must be willing and able to explain the constraints of the methodology, and convince their partners of the necessity of following protocol for the results to be valid. The CBO project director and staff must be willing to compromise with the investigator with regard to research protocol. The researcher must be willing to use and train CBO staff and even residents to do the research. The CBO must be willing to take on extra work, such as completing forms and answering questions. The researcher must be willing to reach compromise with the CBO project director and staff with regard to the clients and community. Sufficient lead time must be allocated to plan, train community staff, and develop the community partners' hypotheses and insights and include them in the questionnaires, interviews, or observation protocols.

Community-researcher teams, which are able to work in this manner and spirit, learn a great deal from each other. As a result, community staff become more sophisticated users and consumers of research. Their skills are enhanced. The organization expands its technical capacity and learns to conduct basic research on its own. They become more competitive for funding because they can better respond to the evaluation and reporting requirements of funders. The researcher learns a great deal more about the community, and is able to collect quality data and test hypotheses that could not otherwise be tested. Researchers' skills in working with communities and CBOs are enhanced, opening the door to future projects and enhanced methods.

Compromising Science?

Some researchers' first reaction to CREPC is that it is a compromise of the scientific model. It is bad enough that the best we can do with hard-to-access populations is get convenience samples. It is a further compromise to make untrained partners central to sample selection, interviews, and interpretation of data. Such a reaction from scientists conveys a fundamental misunderstanding of scientific history and processes. They misunderstand that science is the study, and whenever possible, the measuring of realities. If the physical or social world changes, so must the methods of scientists who wish to study them (Kuhn, 1970; Popper, 1969). The expectation that researchers can rigidly maintain a particular approach to their work across all communities, regardless of their differences, is to ignore reality. Not all communities are the same, and not all groups of people can be accessed or motivated to participate in a study in the same way. Rigid adherence to methods that simply do not work is to ignore the very reality one wished to understand or to simply not appreciate differences as a challenge to science. Here is also where social class, racial, and other bias appear. Only people of higher status than community clients and CBOs can literally walk into a community, claim to be conducting a bias-free study, and then ignore the realities of the people in that community. To not adjust methodology is to expect the community to conform to the higher status scientists' view of reality.

Scientists who rigidly adhere to a model of research show that they do not understand how science advances. The social and behavioral sciences have not advanced by ignoring human realities. In fact, science advances through innovations in methods and theory devised in response to changes in physical and social worlds (Kuhn, 1970). When older techniques for doing research no longer work, the limits of these techniques become apparent. When scientists respond to the limits of their tools and meet the challenges of changing and varied realities, science advances. This has been the case historically. Efforts such as CREPC do not compromise science, but in fact represent extraordinary opportunities to learn more about the social world—to test, refine, and advance existing and new theory.

Some would charge that CREPC further compromises scientists' ability to collect quality data from respondents. They would call into question the reliability and validity of the data and final analysis.

Physical scientists who can precisely measure variables enjoy almost total control over their work. Social and behavioral scientists, who do research in communities, do not have such a luxury and are challenged to devise systematic ways to study social and behavioral phenomena without such controls. It is scientism for a social or behavioral scientist to think that totally controlling who recruits and interviews in the field assures high quality, valid, and reliable data. It does not matter how much control a scientist believes he or she has over data collection; data are seriously compromised if respondents feel that they are "subjects," that the research is more important to the investigator than they are, and that those who conduct the research are not trusted and respected. Under such circumstances, respondents will simply not be available; if found, they will not provide thoughtful responses or take their interview seriously. They will be motivated to sit through the interview only because of the payment.

In contrast, the conditions for a high quality study improve when respondents see participation in a study as an acknowledgement of their humanity and an honest attempt to understand what may be extraordinary about their lives. They will make themselves available and work hard to provide accurate responses to questions. Added incentive is realized if they see that the study is useful and important to the people they work with and receive services from. The bottom line is not who is in control; it is that the best conditions are achieved when respondents are motivated. For hard-to-access populations, the CREPC method is essential.

We Already Know What Is Best for Our Clients

People in community-based agencies also dispute the need for CREPC. Their unique identity may be based on their expertise with clients in their particular service area. Since they provide services, they are also very protective of their clients. A service provider may feel threatened when someone else comes into the agency from the outside, spends a relatively short time with clients, and through the application of science, learns a great deal about them. By sponsoring research, they empower outsiders to comment on and become expert on their clients—a violation of protection and confidence. They may be wary due to concerns that a research project will exploit community clients, compromise an agency's integrity with these clients, or damage their community reputation with funders or the public.

Furthermore, most scientific findings are irrelevant, do not address community-specific concerns, are expensive, or unable to address concerns. Even the best research-based practices may be useless due to inadequate staff or money (Lamb, Greenlick, and McCarty, 1998). Science may seem distant, unfriendly, and not at all relevant to agency work.

A change is needed in the way community-based program service providers think about science. Science is not just for the experts; communities also have a role above and beyond assisting research or acting as research subjects. More important, well-conducted science can help to improve the effectiveness of the services that are offered to clients. Service providers must become more involved in science by contributing their ideas and insights, and then test these ideas along with those of the researcher. Science is most useful to service providers when they have been involved in the planning of research. To ensure client involvement, the service provider must be involved in the day-to-day details of projects. Finally, the service provider needs to be involved in making sense of the findings. At that point, the research is not just for the researchers: it is a vehicle for improving the health of clients. CREPC facilitates such a transition in community thinking and also helps community-based agencies to determine what researchers they will work with. The agency can quickly become very good at distinguishing between those who will work cooperatively with them from those who will not.

A Small Step Forward

As with most innovations in science, CREPC is a progressive and gradual development that was first evident on the margins of a number of disciplines. Kurt Lewin is credited in the late 1940s for devising what was called "action research" to bring theory and application closer together. Action research required close collaboration (Lewin, 1951). A similar development for clinical research (1980) and in AIDS prevention (Binson et al., 1997; Gómez and Goldstein, 1995; Oda, O'Grady, and Strauss, 1994) has been described. For a review of these forerunners of CREPC and descriptions of several other CREPC-like collaborations, see Lamb, Greenlick, and McCarty

Bridging the Gap Between Practice and Research (1998). The principles of CREPC have also been articulated elsewhere (Altman, 1995; Israel et al., 1998). A search of Web sites suggests that there are other collaborative research consortiums underway.*

Aspects of CREPC have been evident since the beginning of efforts to study difficult-to-access communities throughout the past century.

W. E. B. DuBois' *The Philadelphia Negro* (1899) was the first formal study of a problem and difficult-to-access community in the United States. DuBois was introduced to Philadelphia's Seventh Ward by a social services agency. He broadened community trust and acceptance by moving into the community he studied with his family. Prior to World War II, teams of investigators who lived in the immediate community they studied did every major study of community life in the United States. William Lloyd Warner and colleagues moved into different economic sectors of what is now Newburyport, Massachusetts, to produce *The Social Life of a Modern Community* (1941). Muncie, Indiana, was the site of Helen and Robert Lynd's *Middletown* (1929) and *Middletown in Transition* (1937). John Dollard and Dr. Allison Davis' *Deep South* (1941) was conducted in Natchez, Mississippi, and St. Claire Drake and Horace Cayton's *Black Metropolis* (1946) was conducted on Chicago's South Side. The same technique was used in James West's *Plainville, U.S.A.* (1945); in A. B. Hollingshead's *Elmtown's Youth* (1949); and in Hylan Lewis' *Blackways of Kent* (1955). In foreign cultures, anthropologists consider this an essential strategy.

This tradition of fieldwork required immersion in community, establishing trust with informants, and years of observation. Such intense study fell into disuse as cities and towns grew in size and complexity. New statistic-based survey methods were not only cost-effective, but were seen as a more rigorous way to determine the accuracy of complex hypotheses, unlike qualitative studies (Hammersley, 1992; House, 1935). Survey-based studies were less expensive and could be completed in a fraction of the time that it took to complete observational studies (Hammersley, 1992). Anthropologists continue to do community observations, but their work has not drawn

---

*School of Public Health, University of Washington at <http://depts.washington.edu/sphem/academic/comrsch.html>, and the Community Research Network at <http://www.loka.org/crn/index.htm>.

the level of attention that it did during the 1930s and 1940s. Community observation as a form of research almost completely disappeared from mainstream sociology after 1950. Analyses of large national surveys has dominated the sociology flagship journals, pushing those who wish to do qualitative and observational work to the margins of the discipline. The lack of involvement by psychologists in communities is reflected in the efforts of the few community-oriented psychologists to get the mainstream of their discipline interested in communities (Chavis, Stucky, and Wanderman, 1983; Price and Cherniss, 1977; Watters, 1989).

The lack of attention to community in the fields of sociology and psychology created a huge vacuum in our knowledge of community change. As a result, virtually every business and branch of social services have created their own research teams. Now, social workers, city planners, public health workers, criminal justice administrators, nurses, public administrators, and marketing researchers do their own independent research on communities, each with their own journals to report their findings. Since World War II, the federal government has also become increasingly engaged in research. Thus, research has become a huge industry, with specialized and fragmented projects. Community, defined as the complex interconnections between people in their self-defined physical space, became lost amidst categorical agencies, budgets, and research agendas (Bowser, 1998). Community is not just housing, employment, health, transportation, or education—it is how all of these institutions interact and are interconnected. In people's day-to-day lives, all of the different forms of research are connected. However, scientific interest has become focused on data, rather than a more general understanding of people in community. The complexities of people's real lives seem to have been lost in research, whether conducted by academic institutions, government agencies, or social service groups. Meanwhile, thousands of community-based agencies and organizations (CBOs) have emerged in response to critical community needs.

Ironically, the growing recognition of urgent social problems is the result of studies that provided a broad overview based on observation rather than data. Michael Harrington's *The Other America: Poverty in the U.S.* (1969) called attention to poverty in America amidst the postwar affluence. Kenneth Clark's *Dark Ghetto: Dilemmas of Social Power* (1965) provided an inside view of the damaging effects of racial ghettoization. Elliott Liebow's *Tally's Corner: A Study of Negro Streetcorner Men* (1967) portrayed the effects of unemployment on men in community. Carol Stack showed how families survived on welfare and assisted each other in *All Our Kin* (1975). Jonathan Kozol documented the effect of poverty on children in *Rachel and Her Children: Homeless Families in America* (1988). The initial failure of federal, state, and local governments to aggressively address the spread of HIV was documented by Randy Shilts' *And the Band Played On: Politics, People, and the AIDS Epidemic* (1988).

These studies captured the nation's attention and launched government intervention—yet none were based upon highly specialized survey data. What they have in common is a focus on people as they live in their community. This explains why social scientists were unprepared to respond to emerging social problems. It explains why, when the AIDS epidemic hit, social scientists were completely unprepared to mount a systematic prevention effort. When the virus began to spread, scientists were largely ignorant about community and the behaviors of people within them. Sadly, this remains true today.

Only now is there movement to develop research protocols that combine observational study with survey research in community settings (Tashakkori and Teddie, 1998). Urban anthropologists show the necessity to be in the community one studies and to interact with the people one wishes to know more about. Observation and participation is the basis of insight into people's behaviors. Community psychologists have stepped into the role of sociologists by attempting to apply survey research techniques in community settings (Watters, 1989). AIDS prevention necessitated federal research dollars, administered through the National Institute on Drug Abuse, to experiment with combining ethnography with survey research in community studies in the mid-1980s—the National AIDS Demonstration Research (NADR). Almost all but four of the NADR studies were conducted through community-based organizations.

The process of sorting and refining how research should be done in communities is underway. Many scholars—most notably, the U.S. Centers for Disease Control and Prevention—still use the model of "top down," "outside expert," and "full control" research. CREPC is an improvement on this model because it bends techniques of insight and observation with the rigor of survey techniques.

REFERENCES

Agar, M. (1986). *Speaking of Ethnography: Qualitative Research Methods* (Volume 2). Newbury Park, CA: Sage Publications.

Altman, D. (1995). Sustaining interventions in community systems: On the relationship between researchers and communities. *Health Psychology, 14,* 526-536.

Bebbie, E. (1990). *Survey Research Methods.* Belmont: Wadsworth.

Becker, M. and Joseph, J. K. (1988). AIDS and behavior change to reduce risk: A review. *American Journal of Public Health, 78,* 394-410.

Binson, D., Harper, G., Grinstead, O., and Haynes-Sanstad, K. (1997). The center for AIDS prevention studies' collaboration program: An alliance of AIDS scientists and community-based organizations. In P. Nyden, A. Figert, M. Shibley, and D. Borrows (Eds.), *Building Community: Social Science in Action* (pp. 177-189). Thousand Oaks, CA: Pine Forge Press.

Bowser, B. (1994). HIV prevention and African-Americans: A difference of class. In J. P. Van Vugt (Ed.), *AIDS Prevention and Services: Community-Based Research* (pp. 93-108). Westport, CT: Bergin and Garvey.

Bowser, B. (1998). Drug treatment programs and research: The challenge of bidirectionality. In S. Lamb, M. R. Greenlick, and D. McCarty (Eds.), *Bridging the Gap Between Practice and Research: Forging Partnerships with Community-Based Drug and Alcohol Treatment* (pp. 135-146). Washington, DC: National Academy Press.

Carey, J. (1989). *Communications As Culture: Essays on Media and Society.* Boston: Unwin Hyman.

Chavis, D., Stucky, P. E., and Wanderman, A. (1983). Returning basic research to the community: A relationship between scientist and citizen. *American Psychologist, 38,* 424-434.

Clark, K. B. (1965) [1989]. *Dark Ghetto: Dilemmas of Social Power.* Middletown, CT: Wesleyan University Press.

Converse, J. (1987). *Survey Research in the United States: Roots and Emergence, 1890-1960.* Berkeley: University of California Press.

Cox, C. (1994). *Storefront Revolution: Food Co-ops and the Counter-Culture.* New Brunswick, NJ: Rutgers University Press.

Davis, A., Burleigh, B. G., and Gardner, M. R. (1941). *Deep South: A Social Anthropological Study of Caste and Class.* Chicago: University of Chicago Press.

Davis, R. (1995). *The Causal Influence of Perceived Quality of Life on Social Support Among HIV Positive Individuals.* Los Angeles: UCLA.

Denzin, N. and Lincoln, Y. S. (Eds.) (1998). *Strategies of Qualitative Inquiry.* Thousand Oaks, CA: Sage Publications.

Drake, St. Clair and Cayton, H. R. (1946). *Black Metropolis: A Study of Negro Life in a Northern City.* London: J. Cape.

DuBois, W. E. B. (1899) [1967]. *The Philadelphia Negro.* New York: Schocken Books.

Gibson, D. R., McCusker, J., and Chesney, M. (1998). Effectiveness of psychosocial interventions in preventing HIV risk behavior in injecting drug users. *AIDS, 12*(8), 919-1029.

Gómez, C. A. and Goldstein, E. (1995). The HIV prevention evaluation initiative: A model for collaborative evaluation. In D. M. Fetterman, S. J. Kaftaria, and A. Wandersman (Eds.), *Empowerment and Evaluation: Knowledge and Tools for Self-Assessment and Accountability* (pp. 100-122). Thousand Oaks, CA: Sage Publications.

Guba, E. (1990). The alternative paradigm dialog. In E. G. Guba (Ed.), *The Paradigm Dialog* (pp. 17-30). Newbury Park, CA: Sage.

Gubrium, J. and Silverman, D. (Eds.) (1989). *The Politics of Field Research: Sociology Beyond Enlightenment.* Newbury Park, CA: Sage.

Hammersley, M. (1992). *What's Wrong with Ethnography.* London: Routledge Paul.

Harrington, M. (1969). *The Other America: Poverty in the United States.* New York: Macmillan.

Hoffman, E. (1989). *The Politics of Knowledge: Activists Movements in Medicine and Planning.* Albany: State University of New York Press.

Hollingshead, August de Belmont. (1949). *Elmtown's Youth: The Impact of Social Classes on Adolescents.* New York: J. Wiley.

House, F. (1935). Measurement in sociology. *American Journal of Sociology, 40*(1), 1-11.

Hyman, H. and Singer, E. (1991). *Taking Society's Measure: A Personal History of Survey Research.* New York: Russell Sage Foundation.

Israel, B., Schulz, A. J., Parker, E. A., and Becker, A. (1998). Review of community-based research: Assessing partnership approaches to improve public health. *Annual Review of Public Health, 19,* 173-202.

Johnson, J. (1990). *Selecting Ethnographic Informants.* Newbury Park, CA: Sage.

Kozol, J. (1988). *Rachel and Her Children: Homeless Families in America.* New York: Fawcett Columbine.

Kuhn, T. (1970). *The Structure of Scientific Revolutions.* Chicago: The University of Chicago Press.

Lamb, S., Greenlick, M. R., and McCarty, D. (Eds.) (1998). *Bridging the Gap Between Practice and Research: Forging Partnerships with Community-Based Drug and Alcohol Treatment.* Washington, DC: National Academy Press.

Lambert, E., Ashery, R., and Needle, R. (Eds.) (1995). *Qualitative Methods in Drug Abuse and HIV Research* (Volume 157). Rockville, MD: NIDA.

Lewin, K. (1951). *Theory in Social Science: Selected Theoretical Papers.* New York: Harper and Brothers.

Lewis, H. (1955). *Blackways of Kent.* Chapel Hill, NC: University of North Carolina Press.

Liebow, E. (1967). *Tally's Corner: A Study of Negro Streetcorner Men*. Boston: Little, Brown.

Lofland, J. and Lofland, L. H. (1995). *Analyzing Social Settings: A Guide to Qualitative Observation and Analysis* (Third Edition). Belmont, CA: Wadsworth.

Lynd, R. S. and Lynd, H. (1929). *Middletown: A Study in Modern American Culture*. New York: Harcourt, Brace, Jovanovich.

Lynd, R. S. and Lynd, H. (1937). *Middletown in Transition: A Study in Cultural Conflicts*. New York: Harcourt, Brace, and World.

Normand, J., Vlahov, D., and Moses, L. E. (1995). *Preventing HIV Transmission: The Role of Sterile Needles and Bleach*. Washington, DC: National Academy Press.

Oda, D. S., O'Grady, R. S., and Strauss, J. (1994). Collaboration in investigator initiated public health nursing research: University and agency considerations. *Public Health Nursing, 11*, 285-290.

Popper, K. (1969). *The Logic of Scientific Discovery*. New York: Harper.

Price, R. and Cherniss, G. (1977). Training for a new profession: Research as social action. *Professional Psychology, 8*, 222-231.

Shilts, R. (1988). *And the Band Played on: Politics, People, and the AIDS Epidemic*. New York: Penguin Books.

Sloboda, Z. (1998). What we have learned from research about the prevention of HIV transmission among drug abusers. *Public Health Report, 1*, 194.

Stack, C. B. (1975). *All Our Kin: Strategies for Survival in a Black Community*. New York: Harper & Row.

Tashakkori, A. and Teddie, C. (1998). *Mixed Methology: Combining Qualitative and Quantitative Approaches*. Thousand Oaks, CA: Sage Publications.

Van Vugt, J. P. (Ed.) (1994). *AIDS Prevention and Services: Community-Based Research*. Westport, CT: Bergin and Garvey.

Warner, W. L. and Lunt, P. S. (1941) [1973]. *The Social Life of a Modern Community*. Westport, CT: Greenwood Press.

Watters, J. (1989). Observations on the importance of social context in HIV transmission among injection drug users. *Journal of Drug Issues, 19*, 9-29.

Watters, J. (1993). The significance of sampling and understanding hidden populations. *Drugs and Society, 7*, 13-21.

West, J. (1945). *Plainville, U.S.A.* New York: Columbia University Press.

Withers, Carl (1945). *Plainville, U.S.A.* [by] James West [pseud.]. New York: Columbia University Press.

Chapter 2

Collaborative AIDS Research: A Funder's Perspective

Bart K. Aoki
Roger K. Myrick
George F. Lemp
Steve Truax

In the earliest days of the epidemic, AIDS remained in the shadows as the national spotlight and federal resources were directed elsewhere. For a worldwide epidemic that would eventually explode to claim millions of lives and from the perspective of historically disenfranchised communities, funds for research support seemed frustratingly slow in coming. In 1983, in response to delays at the federal level and before the cause of AIDS was known, the state of California entered into a unique partnership with the University of California to support research on AIDS (Das et al., 1991). This partnership, called the Universitywide AIDS Research Program (UARP) grew out of a collaboration of policymakers and a core group of UC faculty when there was no coherent national research policy for addressing the epidemic.

Chapter 2 describes how this university-based research funding entity evolved over time to be a committed advocate of community collaborative AIDS research. Of course, community-science research partnerships have been attempted that predate the unique dynamics of the AIDS epidemic. Thus, in addition to discussing collaborative AIDS research in California and the specific experience of the UARP, we will provide a brief discussion of some of its precedents with an emphasis on the values that have helped shape the collaborative relationships between scientists and community members. Finally, this chapter describes the strategies that UARP developed over the years to foster productive research partnerships and the current challenges that are still to be addressed by the program.

THE VALUES OF COLLABORATIVE RESEARCH

Social scientists have helped shape the process of community research over the past several decades. As a starting point, some social scientists saw *community needs* as central to the research effort. Rather than using theory building as a pursuit in and of itself, these scientists valued the research process as an opportunity to use knowledge in service of meeting these needs. Ultimately, they shared the belief that the quality of social science theory is vastly improved when it is built upon the study of practical problems and in turn becomes a tool for broadening our understanding of specific problems and their larger implications.

Many also perceived the actual research itself as a tool for *social action*. The research was seen as an integral part of a course of action that alters a community and the behavior of its members. The tradition of action research grew out of the early work of Kurt Lewin (1951) who strived to integrate science and practice in research. Key components of the action research cycle included fact-finding, action, and evaluation (Ketterer, Price, and Politser, 1980). In this process, descriptive research to gather initial data on the nature of the problem was a step in a cycle that led to the formulation of community level goals, which were then implemented through concerted action to help solve community problems. The final step in any action research was an evaluation of the success of the community intervention so that the cycle could begin anew.

Last, many scientists believed that community research should result in *useful products*. This went beyond the publication of results in academic journals: new program manuals, improved service structures, strengthened and expanded skills for the staff of community organizations, and new systems for program evaluation were all practical products highly valued by action-oriented community researchers. Understandably, products were seen as even more useful if they were also adopted and used over time within communities. Researchers and public health agencies had long recognized the elusiveness of going from successful pilot programs to widespread adoption of new interventions. Although part of the difficulty of disseminating new innovations could be attributed to the unique character of each locality, a sense of community ownership and investment in the change process were also seen as part of the necessary foundation (Blakeley et al., 1987). Meaningful collaborative partnerships with community participants were seen, in turn, as integral to the sense of community ownership and the eventual likelihood that pilot programs would be sustained (Altman, 1995).

Despite these common values, the degree and actual success of collaboration between scientists and the community have varied considerably. This variability has sometimes been influenced by the actual research approach or methodology being used (D'Aunno and Price, 1984). Methods aimed at documenting the occurrence of a particular social or public health problem through direct surveys or through the analyses of other problem indicators did not necessitate a high degree of collaboration. On the other hand, methods that called for the delivery of different types of interventions or for the direct participation and observation by researchers required the establishment of much more meaningful collaborative relationships in order to be feasible and ultimately successful.

Despite the traditional dictates of discipline and methodology, active and meaningful *collaborations* between scientists and those who participated in their research came to be seen as a dimension critical to the success of action-oriented research. As a result, numerous attempts at research collaborations were conceptualized and studied (Baker et al., 1999; Cousins and Early, 1992; Hatch et al., 1993; Oda, O'Grady, and Strauss, 1994). Because these attempts often encountered enormous difficulties, this process also enabled researchers to identify additional factors critical to community collaboration. These included acknowledging the real difference between community input and active community involvement; attending to mutual trust and respect; acknowledging and honoring different agendas; and being aware of transitions and points of stress in the partner organizations. During this era, enormous amounts of public resources were also being allocated to support collaborative research demonstrations, particularly for the prevention of substance abuse, mental disorders, and the social and public health problems of the 1970s and 1980s (Baldwin, 1999; Campbell, 1997; Fawcett et al., 1995). As with previous attempts, these efforts also met with varying degrees of success.

The current collaborative research program at the Universitywide AIDS Research Program is a direct outgrowth of the numerous attempts over the past three decades to fully realize the concept of community collaborative research. It is based on the premise that for research collaborations to be truly successful, the goals of both researchers and communities must be equally served. For this reason, UARP has defined community collaborative research as projects that involve the joint and equal participation of researchers and community members from the inception of the effort, including conceiving of the goals, the design, the development and implementation, and the ultimate evaluation of its project's success.

CHALLENGES TO COMMUNITY COLLABORATIONS AND HIV PREVENTION RESEARCH

Community collaboration and an action-oriented focus of research have been particularly important for HIV prevention research for two primary reasons. First, HIV has historically impacted disenfranchised, underserved communities that lack access to mainstream political power and health care opportunities, greatly affecting their response to HIV. Second, HIV has presented boundless challenges to social science researchers because of the complexities of social/sexual identity and behaviors—particularly those that are extremely difficult to measure and assess using traditional research methodologies. Although the need has been great, collaboration between these two groups has been unusually difficult because of the volatile and highly politicized context of HIV.

The politicization of HIV/AIDS occurred during its initial stages through government inaction and political- and media-savvy activists' response to that inaction. The early discourse about HIV/AIDS was framed as a battle between disenfranchised communities who were dying because of a lack of access to resources and the powerful political and medical constituencies who were in control of those resources. In many ways, the HIV/AIDS epidemic catapulted critical social and public health issues into a new light, one that demanded a collaborative response from multiple stakeholders with distinct needs and political interests.

Collaboration has been difficult on one level because powerful research institutions have often been positioned outside of the real-life circumstances of affected and infected communities whose immediate needs are served by community-based organizations (CBOs). The lingering result has been the creation of a wide gulf between groups who need one another's expertise and access, but who find themselves in separate philosophical and political camps.

Researchers and community providers are also faced with significant material differences that affect their ability to collaborate successfully.

For example, many community organizations' main focus is on providing services and prevention education to populations affected by HIV and a number of life-challenging circumstances. Service providers measure their success in terms of the extent to which the organization responds to the dynamic and extensive needs of historically underserved communities, which requires a great deal of flexibility on the part CBOs. Further informing the context in which CBOs operate is a constant struggle to maintain operations in the face of extremely limited resources, including ongoing staff turnover and budgetary limitations. Although funders often encourage or require CBOs to carry out research activities, funds are not always provided to support such efforts. As a result, CBOs can experience difficulty finding the time, money, or staff necessary to conduct scientific research on prevention programs. CBOs may also be reluctant to embrace certain types of research—such as evaluation—because they may be perceived as a threat to programs that have historical significance or provide funding for the organization.

In addition, the methodological rigor required for scientific research can actually interfere with the provision of services and prevention education, which is the CBO's primary function. Research operations can be seen as burdensome, and methodologies can be perceived as an impediment to working with target populations, who may view research agendas and operations with a great deal of suspicion.

Finally, CBOs are not always included as equal partners in the planning and implementation of research projects; as a result, a CBO may feel as though it is being subjected to research rather than participating in the project as a partner with equal value and necessary investment (Reed and Collins, 1994). If the CBO is not involved in planning, the intervention may not be responsive to the unique environment of the CBO and the needs of its target populations. The outcome can be a research project that fails to achieve the goals of either the researcher or the service provider and works against the purpose of community-based, action-focused research.

On the other hand, researchers working in academic institutions face their own unique set of challenges. For example, scientific researchers have a primary purpose of generating new knowledge through scientifically sound research. Researchers' success is measured through grant awards and publications that are the result of the rigorous application of the scientific method, criteria that may mean little to community organizations attempting to meet immediate survival needs of target populations.

Of course, funding plays a key role in the success of any research effort, and differences in financial capacity and operations between research and community organizations can create a significant impediment to the success of collaboration. For example, by their very nature, research projects tend to be long-term endeavors that require reliable, relatively stable funding. Funding for researchers typically comes from both university and government funding streams and tends to be more stable and long-term than budgets of CBOs, which are often funded through yearly donations, short-term grants, and government reimbursement programs. High CBO staff turnover and the tenuous, short-term nature of funding can undermine long-term project stability.

Although community organizations are at their best when they are able to remain flexible and respond to changing needs of target populations and fluctuations in resources, scientific researchers must maintain a great degree of control over research environments and target populations in order to ensure the methodological rigor of research. Only by controlling for external influences can scientists ensure that the research outcomes and target populations' responses are due to the impact of the prevention intervention. From the researcher's perspective, the dynamic and community-driven nature of the CBO can pose a significant methodological challenge, particularly with respect to random sampling procedures; assignment of subjects to control and intervention groups; systematic, long-term data collection; and the use of research instruments and consent forms (Binson et al., 1997).

Researchers must also be prepared to conduct extensive training with staff, including all project participants, which can be an extremely time-consuming task and may involve initially persuading staff of the importance and relevance of research efforts.

On one level, collaborations are expensive, time consuming, and difficult to effectively implement (Human Interaction Research Institute, 1998), and in many ways run counter to the operational procedures and identities of both types of organizations. Because of distinct research and community cultures, initial efforts at collaboration are often unsuccessful. Research institutions tend to focus on generating data, while community organizations are often left without enhanced capacity for research, or useful results from research efforts that could be used in practical ways for improvements in prevention programs.

OPPORTUNITIES OFFERED BY COLLABORATIVE HIV PREVENTION RESEARCH

Since the early 1990s, AIDS service organizations and HIV prevention researchers have been responding to challenges by looking toward collaboration as a way of using scientific research to improve HIV prevention efforts in community settings. Ultimately, it has been the course of the epidemic itself and a resulting acknowledgement of mutual value and need that has brought HIV prevention researchers and community advocates together. Without the scientific expertise that researchers offer in the design and evaluation of interventions, community organizations cannot be sure that their prevention programs are making a difference. Researchers can offer evidence of why programs do or do not result in intended outcomes, so that interventions can be enhanced and made more effective (Reed and Collins, 1994). In turn, without the access to populations that community organizations offer, social and behavioral scientists interested in HIV prevention research often remain separated from the disenfranchised communities where risky behaviors are occurring and where prevention science and its application can be advanced. For researchers, such collaborations can result in new research questions and direct application of science (Reed and Collins, 1994). Collaborative research can also provide access to funding for both the CBO and researcher that might not otherwise be available and ultimately strengthen the CBO's capacity for sustaining interventions (Human Interaction Research Group, 1998), the primary goal of action-focused, collaborative research.

In recent years, collaborative prevention research in AIDS has progressed in a number of research centers around the country (Haynes-Sanstad et al., 1999; Hunter, Wyuche, and Warne, 1998; Schensul, 1999). Notably, successful collaborations have not been the result of the logical development of scientific and community interaction. Rather, successful collaborations have most often been the result of researchers who come from infected and affected communities who are able to bridge research and community perspectives in ways that empower community organizations to use research to strengthen and improve HIV prevention efforts and the lives of people who have been disproportionately and heavily impacted by HIV. This marks a shift in the purpose of research—making the needs of the community paramount. This shift would not have occurred without members of infected and affected communities taking the lead in rethinking what the purpose and use of HIV prevention research should be.

In California, two highly successful collaborative efforts—one funded and implemented through a University of California San Francisco (UCSF) and California Department of Health Services/Office of AIDS (OA) partnership and one through a collaboration among UCSF, Bay Area community organizations, and Northern California Grantmakers —helped lay the groundwork for collaborative research in California as well as the rest of the nation. Collaborating partners from these projects have drawn several conclusions about successful strategies for conducting community research.

Organizations must identify common goals from the outset, such as the successful procurement of prevention research funding and the enhancement of prevention interventions. Obviously, funding organizations such as UARP can play a critical role in the establishment of incentives, common goals, and opportunities for collaborative partners. Organizations must also recognize each other's organizational capabilities and accommodate these in designing the collaboration; there must be mutual agreement on respective contributions, roles, timelines, and accountability—issues that must also include substantive input from the target population (Fox, 1995; Reed and Collins, 1994).

As they plan for collaboration, organizations must educate themselves about each other's organizational needs and operational procedures, which will have an impact on the collaboration, and develop responsive strategies that will enhance interaction. For example, researchers must establish a substantive connection with the community organization and target communities, which means regular contact and communication and the realization that the CBO's clients' needs are of utmost importance (Binson et al., 1997).

Researchers must also be cognizant of the dynamic nature of CBOs and develop a certain flexibility regarding research design to ensure that research is relevant for the organization, helping it to achieve its goals. One successful collaborator recommended the development of primary and secondary research elements, including research questions and instruments, that would meet the researchers' methodological requirements and simultaneously offer immediate and needed feedback to the CBO about its prevention efforts (Binson et al., 1997). In fact, all aspects of research design must remain responsive to the unique needs and context of the CBO and its target populations.

Likewise, CBOs must respond to the researchers' need for methodological rigor and must become familiar with evaluation research design and use. CBOs must fully buy into the research endeavor and recognize its applicability to strengthening prevention efforts. For both the researcher and the community partner, each must reprioritize work to incorporate the needs of the other (Gómez and Goldstein, 1995).

Above all, successful collaborators have found that open communication is essential; organizations must communicate constructively and frequently to share ideas, work through challenges, plan for responses, and ultimately to maintain trust.

In summary, successful collaboration requires that research and community organizations work as partners from the outset, with community empowerment as a primary goal. This requires the active involvement of both partners in defining research questions, agreeing on practical methodology, and developing a shared understanding of the use of research.

FUNDING FOR COMMUNITY RESEARCH
ON AIDS: UARP

UARP's Early Experience

Particularly important to the progress of HIV prevention research are the funding opportunities designed to enhance social science and community collaborative partnerships. In response to this need and in the context of the second wave of HIV—when the disease's impact on disenfranchised communities increased visibly—the UARP moved toward what would become the Collaborative AIDS Prevention Research Initiative. The process and events that led to UARP's Collaborative AIDS Prevention Research Initiative can be understood as an extended process of collaboration among differing constituencies and organizations, characterized by all of its pitfalls and challenges.

By the late 1980s, a growing realization emerged that the virus was proving to be a formidable foe, that advances in biomedical science were likely to be incremental at best, and that a cure lay far in the distant future. However, despite an increasing consensus that prevention was key to slowing the epidemic, and the increasing need to incorporate social and behavioral research into prevention planning and evaluation, divergent interests seemed to impede any significant shift of UARP's funding toward this end. Membership of the UARP Task Force on AIDS—UARP's advisory group—by the mid-to-late 1980s consisted primarily of biomedical scientists who, understandably, made funding recommendations consistent with their experience and perspectives.

In 1987, under increasing pressure by community members and social scientists from around the state, the program acted to form an ad hoc Committee for Behavioral Research on AIDS, chaired by Dr. Ray Catalano. Despite this concrete action and the efforts of the committee, the process of changing minds and changing program priorities proceeded in what was probably perceived by other stakeholders at an intolerably slow and imperceptible pace. This prompted these stakeholders, both community members and social scientists from around the state, to seek assistance from then State Assemblyman Tom Hayden. As chair of the Assembly Subcommittee on Higher Education, he held the power to recommend hearings aimed at influencing the priorities of the University of California and UARP and, at the urging of these constituents, he exercised his authority. Hearings were held in the state capitol in May 1988 to look into the extent of UARP's funding of social and behavioral science research.

As a result of the hearings, the state's Joint Legislative Budget Committee issued sixteen formal recommendations directing the UARP to increase its investment in research into the social and behavioral aspects of AIDS. Included were recommendations to strengthen the representation of social/behavioral scientists as full participants in the AIDS Task Force and three separate recommendations urging increased levels of collaboration with community-based organizations in research efforts and in the dissemination of research findings. In response to these recommendations, the program took several immediate steps. In November 1989, UARP issued a comprehensive request for applications on social/behavioral science research in AIDS. To further stimulate activity in prevention, education, and community research in AIDS, the Task Force also initiated a predoctoral training grant program for educating students in social sciences. Finally, the Task Force set a goal to fund social science grant applications at an amount equal to the basic and clinical sciences.

Between 1990 and 1993, the Task Force also supported a series of conferences on these issues. Three of them were focused specifically on developing collaboration in AIDS research and service delivery. Geoffey Reed and Barry Collins (1994), researchers at UCLA at the time, described how an advocacy coalition of people living with AIDS (PWAs) confronted organizers about their exclusion from the planning process for these conferences. The organizers, primarily UC faculty, were forced to acknowledge that, in a conference about collaboration, few CBO representatives had been invited or otherwise encouraged to participate. Identified PWAs had not been involved in any formal way, and organizers came to realize that they had "unintentionally participated in disempowerment of people living with HIV and AIDS" (Reed and Collins, 1994, p. 72). Consequently, the last conference in the series included members of HIV-infected and affected communities in all phases of the conference. A "three communities model" of collaboration among researchers, community-based organizations, and persons living with HIV/AIDS emerged. It was based on the idea that HIV intervention research and service delivery "should include constructive collaboration among these three communities throughout all phases of research and practice" (Reed and Collins, 1994, p. 70). Consistent with this model, conference participants conceived of an active role for federal or other funding agencies through their use of economic incentives (i.e., grant funding) to foster collaboration in AIDS research.

In fall 1993, following on the heels of achieving what appeared to be a broad consensus about the necessity of collaborative AIDS research, the UARP initiated discussions with the California Department of Health Services, Office of AIDS (OA) on how UARP might collaborate with that agency to foster these activities in California. Although the initial discussions kept in mind the clear distinction between the two agencies, i.e., UARP's mission of supporting research and the Office of AIDS in prevention and education services, these differences would ultimately prove fatal to this first attempt at interagency collaboration. Many hours of planning and negotiation were spent in crafting a collaborative agreement that would account for the organizational differences in mission, values, culture, and operating authority and policies. At one point in the process it appeared an agreement had been reached that would establish a "full and equal partnership" of the two state entities charged with different aspects of the AIDS epidemic in California.

Similar to many other attempts at collaboration by entities with divergent goals and values, however, this first attempt was unsuccessful. Late in 1994, negotiations broke off after more than a year of intensive effort by committed staff and community members. At that time differences in how the collaborative partnership would share authority and decision making and how this could be reconciled with contracting procedures and precedents seemed an insurmountable obstacle. However, as a result of both parties' commitment to the concept, the UARP Task Force decided to proceed independently with a collaborative AIDS prevention research initiative, funded solely by the resources of UARP. The UARP's subsequent Collaborative AIDS Prevention Research Initiative issued its first Request for Applications (RFA) in 1995.

UARP's Initial Funding
for Collaborative Prevention Research

As a funder, UARP's prevention research initiative reflected a recognition of the need for a research funding mechanism that would provide resources for collaboration in a way that substantively united research and community organizations, encouraging recognition and consideration of the strengths, needs, identities, and cultures of each, and establishing requirements for common goals and operational strategies that would bring the organizations together as partners. The goals of UARP's 1995 RFA were to encourage and enable good science and to empower community organizations to enhance their prevention programs, ultimately resulting in the decline of HIV infections in California.

UARP's initial collaborative funding project included several strategies designed to respond to the problems with collaboration and to ensure effective, equal partnerships in the collaborative process.

First, the UARP designed a Request for Applications (RFA) whose purpose incorporated the needs of both research and community organizations. The RFA's stated purpose was to,

> foster prevention research collaboration between scientific researchers and AIDS service organizations/local government agencies, so that AIDS prevention strategies can be evaluated, innovative methods can be tested, investigators can share theoretical and methodological insights, and the CBO/agency can develop procedures and infrastructure for collecting data needed for in-house and statewide monitoring of prevention efforts. (UARP, 1994, p. 4)

This purpose combines the research priorities of scientists with the CBO's need for monitoring prevention programs, thereby unifying organizations by establishing a common goal of collaborative prevention research.

The UARP (1994) further ensured equal collaboration by framing evaluation and review criteria in the RFA in a way that guarded against the misuse of the relationship by either party:

> CBOs are reminded that the use of the principal investigators (PIs) simply to gain access to a new source of funds for service provision is not acceptable. PIs are reminded that use of a CBO simply to gain access to a study population and recruit subjects is not acceptable. Data collection and other activities must by conducted collaboratively for an application to be competitive. (p. 5)

The RFA also required substantial documentation of the collaborative relationship in the application for the RFA. Requirements included evidence of a collaborative team approach to research; shared vision and goals with the CBO; researcher experience working with CBOs; CBO-researcher collaboration from the inception of development, implementation, and evaluation of an innovative intervention or the evaluation of an existing intervention; a detailed explanation of all collaborative arrangements, including financial management, data collection, data analysis, training, technical assistance, protection of human subjects, and dissemination of research results; responsibilities and roles of each partner; any provisions for regular discussions or meetings; and methods for conflict resolution and problem solving.

These guidelines served as the criteria on which review decisions were made, ensuring that the projects selected represented not only strong scientific efforts with a high likelihood of success, but projects that were conceptualized, implemented, and evaluated on the basis of the collaborative vision, interaction, and operations of the two organizations.

To ensure successful, collaborative implementation of the grantees' projects, the UARP program officer convened a meeting at the outset with the principal investigators and their CBO collaborators, members of the UARP Task Force, and other UARP investigators who were conducting community-based prevention research to discuss and offer guidance for all projects funded. The purpose of the meeting was to ensure that, as projects got underway, equal partnerships were in place that accommodated and empowered both organizations, their goals, and operations, and included recommendations for enhancements of critical project elements such as research design and methodology and development of CBO infrastructure for research. UARP also made use of this initial meeting to help identify ways that it could provide needed support to the collaborative efforts.

Finally, the UARP required that successful grantees form a consortium which met quarterly to coordinate and evaluate their research results with the ultimate aim of developing effective AIDS prevention intervention programs that could be adopted and implemented by AIDS organizations throughout the state. The consortium meetings included speakers from community and research organizations with experience in collaboration who addressed relevant issues and topics;

workshops that focused on research criteria and data elements that could be used by other collaborative projects statewide; technical assistance; and small and large group discussions of challenges and successes with the collaborative process.

The first community collaborative prevention RFA was offered in 1995, became a regular part of UARP's funding mechanisms in 1996, and has resulted in the funding of a total of twelve collaborative projects focusing on prevention interventions and evaluations that respond to HIV/AIDS in California, many of which are detailed in this book. As a whole, UARP's collaborative initiative has been highly successful. Projects not only resulted in scientifically-grounded evaluations of prevention programs critical to the state's HIV/AIDS response, but they have also resulted in the wide dissemination of information on collaborative research, improvement of prevention efforts, and research-capacity building in CBOs. The projects have also enabled the development of collaborative relationships between research and community organizations that UARP is using as a model for current and future research and funding opportunities.

UARP's Recent Collaborative Prevention Evaluation Funding Initiative

In addition to the creation of a permanent, institutionalized mechanism for funding community collaborations, UARP has gone on to establish a prevention evaluation funding initiative through the long sought-after partnership with the State Office of AIDS (OA). Four years after the first attempt, in what could be seen as a tribute to the commitment and effort of those involved with the first aborted efforts, the university and OA came together again, and this time, in 1998, were able to reach an agreement that expanded the collaborative prevention research efforts and capacity of both organizations. One of the greatest challenges facing this effort was ensuring that research was used in a way that directly addressed the impact of HIV on public health needs specific for California. Toward that end, the UARP and the OA initiated an interagency agreement designed to develop and implement a collaborative evaluation strategy for HIV prevention and planning activities in California that would equalize the roles of researchers and community advocates. To be successful, both parties kept their eyes on the overarching goal of strengthening California AIDS prevention programs as they impact the state's high-priority populations and communities, and made extraordinary efforts to extend themselves to understand and work with each other's priorities and constraints. The interagency agreement provides an equal degree of autonomy, control, and clearly defined roles for both the UARP and OA, with OA functioning as the funder and UARP functioning as the scientific consultant and peer review and grant administrator on the project. As with the researcher/CBO projects, the relationship between the funding entities had to be defined in such a way that allowed each to function consistently with existing organizational goals, identities, and cultures.

As part of the interagency agreement, UARP and OA issued an RFA for collaborative, multiyear research projects to evaluate prevention interventions throughout the state. In preparation for the RFA, the UARP convened the Prevention Evaluation Advisory Committee (PEAC), comprised of leaders from California's research institutions, AIDS service organizations, CDC, and NIH representatives, and members of infected and affected communities, to advise the Universitywide AIDS Task Force and the OA. This again illustrates an effort by UARP and OA to include a large number of stakeholders—including scientists, public health experts, providers, and consumers—in the decision-making and planning process for community collaborative prevention evaluation efforts statewide, a clear indication of the impact earlier collaborations had on the operational procedures of both organizations. Increasingly, more and more voices were being included in the planning and implementation of HIV prevention research efforts, and the distinct goals of California researchers, providers, and consumer advocates were being galvanized around the central purpose of promoting prevention research based on community needs, social action, and the production of useful products.

The RFA was released in November 1998, followed by four bidders' conferences held throughout the state. As a point of interest, the most common concern raised at these conferences was that several community organizations expressed the need to be more connected with research networks, indicating a desire on the part of the CBOs for scientific evaluation of programs, and a feeling of limited access to research opportunities. UARP responded by facilitating connections among groups and individuals with similar backgrounds and interests, but the need for networking remains significant.

For the 1998 RFA, UARP developed a number of enhancements to its original collaborative funding mechanism and review process in an attempt to ensure an equal partnership between participating organizations. First, the new RFA treated both the community and scientific participants as PIs for the project, shifting away from the PI/subcontractor relationship used in the 1995 and 1997 mechanisms. In fact, the 1998 mechanism disbursed money directly to both the research and community-based organizations. The application also required identical information and documentation for each collaborator; in some ways the application treated each organization distinctly in terms of budget, documentation of experience, and operational procedures, thereby maintaining the individual integrity and identity of both collaborative partners. However, a critical component of the application was the documentation of specific collaborative activities and designated roles and responsibilities, establishing common goals and clear accountability for all aspects of the research project at the outset. The result was a funding mechanism that created equal opportunities for both partners to use their individual and collective value to advance prevention evaluation research.

As with all UARP grant applications, a committee combining research and CBO experts reviewed the applications received in response to the RFA. However, unlike the traditional committee make-up which includes a majority of scientific reviewers who function as primary readers and a minority of community reviewers who serve as secondary and tertiary readers, the review committee for the new collaborative mechanism was unique in its composition. It had an equal mix of scientific and community reviewers who all served as primary and secondary readers, thereby creating a collaborative experience and equalizing of voices in the review process itself.

Following the review and awarding of funding, grant recipients formed a consortium that meets regularly to develop common evaluation criteria, data elements, and research strategies that can be used to assess the effectiveness of prevention efforts throughout California. The consortium represents the union of public health and scientific research efforts that facilitate work on specific projects, build capacity within CBOs for research, and, ultimately, move research initiatives toward the development of statewide guidelines for collaborative prevention evaluation research.

UARP's most recent experience offers several important insights into both collaborative research and the funding process for such research. For instance, while UARP had been careful to ensure the establishment of collaborative partnerships and a focus on the diverse needs of Californians through its application and review process, it was clear that even greater guidance was needed in certain areas. For instance, more front-end technical assistance was needed for both community representatives and research scientists in the development of collaborative research projects and proposals; in several instances, applicants seemed to struggle with establishing equal partnerships between parties, and often resorted to traditional roles that actually worked against collaboration. Even in some successful applications, there tended to be an unequal distribution of resources and a resistance toward open, mutual, and direct communication, negotiation, and collaboration. In addition, there was the sense on the part of the scientific and community "peer" reviewers that they needed more specific information on key definitions and concepts regarding collaboration, and on their roles as reviewers. As a new process, reviewers were not always comfortable considering both scientific and community perspectives—although each reviewer was selected for his or her extensive experience in both roles.

Finally, while all applicants targeted high-risk populations in their applications, the strongest applicants focused on urban locations that had been subjected to a great deal of research scrutiny. The result was a lack of research devoted to rural areas and other underresearched locations and populations, indicating a need for targeted funding opportunities that would respond to the diversity of California even more substantively and strategically.

One of the greatest challenges for the collaboration between UARP and OA as funders came to light following the review and prior to the determination of the initial funding line. The top three ranked applications—which absorbed the majority of the allocated funds for the project—clustered around one research institution and were located in one urban area. In order to merge the scientific merit rankings (as determined by UARP's review process) with the diverse needs of a state the size of California (as identified by the OA), UARP and OA negotiated budget recommendations for PIs that allowed for the funding of a fourth highly ranked and meritorious application that was focused on an additional research institution and geographic location. The result was the funding of four highly meritorious projects that offer statewide significance for California's HIV prevention efforts. However, the results also point out that scientific merit and statewide focus do not always coincide; in a state with the size and diversity of California, ensuring this is crucial. Plans for future collaborative funding efforts include the offering of a series of statewide technical assistance workshops for applicants and a possible targeted RFA that would focus efforts on underresearched areas of need in specific geographic locations throughout the state.

CONCLUSION

Interestingly, many of the challenges and opportunities that researchers and CBOs face in doing collaborative research and prevention are also faced by funding organizations when they collaborate. Only by accommodating each other's needs, clearly defining respective roles, expectations, and accountability, and establishing and maintaining open lines of communication, will the collaborative efforts of any organization succeed.

The collaborative projects in this book represent collaboration at its best—research and community experts working together to meet challenges and achieve critical prevention and research goals. These projects also illustrate the advances that are possible when funders provide support for innovative science and public health endeavors that realize their greatest potential when efforts are joined.

REFERENCES

Altman, D. (1995). Sustaining interventions in community systems: On the relationship between researchers and communities. *Health Psychology, 14,* 526-536.

Baker, E., Homan, S., Schonhoff, R., and Kreuter, M. (1999). Principles of practice for academic/practice/community research partnerships. *American Journal of Preventive Medicine, 16*(3 Supplement), 86-93.

Baldwin, J. (1999). Conducting drug abuse prevention research in partnership with Native American communities: Meeting challenges through collaborative approaches. *Drugs and Society, 14,* 77-92.

Binson, D., Harper, G., Grinstead, O., and Haynes-Sanstad, K. (1997). The center for AIDS prevention studies' collaboration program: An alliance of AIDS scientists and community-based organizations. In A.F.P. Nyden, M. Shibley, and D. Borrows (Eds.), *Building Community: Social Science in Action* (pp. 177-189). Thousand Oaks, CA: Pine Forge Press.

Blakeley, C., Mayer, J.P., Gottschalk, R.G., Schmitt, N., Davidson, W.S., Roitman, D.B., and Emshoff, J.G. (1987). The fidelity-adaptation debate: Implications for the implementation of public sector social programs. *American Journal of Community Psychology, 15,* 253-268.

Campbell, J. (1997). How consumers/survivors are evaluating the quality of psychiatric care. *Evaluation Review, 21,* 357-363.

Cousins, J.E. and Early, L.M. (1992). The case for participatory evaluation. *Educational Evaluation and Policy Analysis, 14,* 397-418.

Das, N., Hopper, C.L., Jencks, M., and Silva, J. (1991). A University of California state-supported AIDS research award program—a unique state and university partnership in AIDS research. *Journal of Clinical Immunology, 11,* 65-73.

D'Aunno, T.P. and Price, R.H. (1984). The context and objectives of community research. In R.K. Heller, Price, S. Reinharz, S. Riger, and A. Wandersman (Eds.), *Psychology and Community Change: Challenges of the Future* (pp. 51-67). Pacific Grove, CA: Brooks/Cole Publishing Co.

Fawcett, S., Paine-Andrews, A., Francisco, V.T., Schultz, J.A., Richter, K.P., Lewis, R.K., Williams, E., Harris, K.J., Berkley, J.Y., and Fisher, J.L. (1995). Using empowerment theory in collaborative partnerships for community health and development. *American Journal of Community Psychology, 23,* 677-697.

Fox, J. (1995). Collaborative research pitfalls examined: Ethics colloquium outlines key issues researchers need to consider when embarking on collaborative enterprises. *American Society for Microbiology News, 61,* 517-519.

Gómez, C. and Goldstein, E. (1995). The HIV prevention evaluation initiative: A model for collaborative evaluation. In D.M. Fetterman, S.J. Kaftarian, and A. Wandersman (Eds.), *Empowerment and Evaluation: Knowledge and Tools for Self-Assessment and Accountability* (pp. 100-122). Thousand Oaks, CA: Sage Publications.

Hatch, J., Moss, N., Saran, A., Presley-Cantrell, L., and Mallory, C. (1993). Community research: Partnership in Black communities. *American Journal of Preventive Medicine, 9*(6 Supplement), 27-31.

Haynes-Sanstad, K., Stall, R., Goldstein, E., Everett, W., and Brousseau, R. (1999). Collaborative community research consortium: A model for HIV prevention. *Health Education and Behavior, 26,* 171-184.

Human Interaction Research Institute (1998). San Francisco Bay Area HIV/AIDS prevention and evaluation initiative: Lesson for funders, nonprofits and evaluators. San Francisco: Northern California Grantmakers AIDS Task Force.

Hunter, J., Wyuche, K., and Warne, P. (1998). Evaluation of a researcher-community collaboration: The development of an HIV Prevention Curriculum for

Gay/Lesbian/Bisexual Youth. Paper presented at the Twelfth World AIDS Conference, Geneva, Switzerland, July 9.

Ketterer, R., Price, R.H., and Politser, P.E. (1980). The action research paradigm. In R.H. Price and Politser, P.E. (Eds.), *Evaluation and Action in the Social Environment.* New York: Academic Press.

Oda, D., O'Grady, R.S., and Strauss, J. (1994). Collaboration in investigator initiated public health nursing research: University and agency considerations. *Public Health Nursing, 11,* 285-290.

Reed, G. and Collins, B.E. (1994). Mental health research and service delivery: A three communities model. *Psychosocial Rehabilitation Journal, 17,* 70-81.

Schensul, J. (1999). Organizing community research partnerships in the struggle against AIDS. *Health Education and Behavior, 26,* 266-283.

Universitywide AIDS Research Program (UARP) (1994). Request for applications. Oakland, CA: UARP.

Chapter 3

Preventing AIDS Among Injectors and Sex Workers

Gloria Lockett
Carla Dillard-Smith
Benjamin P. Bowser

The city of Oakland and Alameda County have one of the highest HIV infection rates in the state of California and these rates are continuing to climb (Reardon, 1994; Watters, Bluthental, and Kral, 1995). If this uncontrolled epidemic is going to be slowed, it will have to happen through CAL-PEP, which is the primary and largest HIV prevention outreach service in the East Bay.

The California Prevention Education Program (CAL-PEP) does street outreach to people at high risk of HIV infection in San Francisco and primarily the East Bay, bringing services directly to clients where they congregate and engage in high-risk behavior. To find clients, outreach workers go to street corners and alleys, abandoned buildings, crack houses, shooting galleries, check cashing centers, soup kitchens, homeless camps, and single occupancy hotels.

CAL-PEP reaches clients in the late evenings and early mornings, offering HIV prevention education and materials such as bleach to clean syringes and free condoms. They also give referrals to social services, housing, medical care, and provide on-site medical care from a county health van. These are standard activities for comprehensive HIV/AIDS outreach programs (Ashery et al., 1995; Astemborski et al., 1994). The CAL-PEP staff has gained a reputation for their dedicated work, creating a relationship of trust and rapport with clients. Many CAL-PEP staff have moved on to direct other social service programs. Others have enrolled in graduate and medical school.

For a "front-line" prevention organization such as CAL-PEP, two questions are of utmost importance. First: how effective are their services? Second: can their work be improved? The absence of rigorous evaluation has been a barrier to stable funding, preventing the CAL-PEP outreach model from getting wider attention.

BEGINNING OF COLLABORATION

The inception of the CAL-PEP collaboration began with conversations, over several years, between CAL-PEP director, Gloria Lockett, and Benjamin Bowser, a sociologist at California State University, Hayward. After various AIDS conferences, they discussed the importance of a CAL-PEP evaluation. They also agreed that a scientific approach to prevention research must be community based to have relevance to clients' lives. An opportunity for Lockett and Bowser to address both concerns appeared in the fall of 1996 with funding of a Collaborative Research Grant from the University of California University-wide AIDS Research Program (UARP). How was a community-based CAL-PEP evaluation created? How was the science improved? First of all, it was not presumed that all of the knowledge for understanding CAL-PEP services was already in the scientific literature. Second, CAL-PEP as an organization and staff were neither subjects to be analyzed, nor were they just a field site to gain access to HIV high-risk subjects.

The starting assumption was that the CAL-PEP outreach staff had insight about their clients that was equally as important as scientists' more technical knowledge—and that both sets of expertise should be utilized. A second assumption was that CAL-PEP services are not one-dimensional or straightforward. To better understand their services, it was important to work with the staff to better understand what they do, how they do it, and what their goals are. Finally, it was recognized that the project needed the cooperation and involvement of CAL-PEP outreach staff to locate both clients and nonclients, so the two groups of at-risk people could be compared—then re-recruited, and compared again, one year later.

Fulfillment of these goals entailed an apparent contradiction: first, the evaluation had to be independent of CAL-PEP staff so as not to be biased. At the same time, it had to be endorsed by CAL-PEP staff so they would share their knowledge of what they do and help the interview team to get full access to their clients.

Defining the Research Questions

At the outset of the evaluation project, the CAL-PEP staff was very clear: They were suspicious of research, believing that a lot of research had already been done on their clients and had been of little use in improving their work. Researchers had come, published their papers, then gone—leaving little of lasting value. Furthermore, the staff was hesitant about an evaluation of their work. They considered it a waste of time or just another administrative burden. It might uncover what they were doing wrong. They also were wary that outsiders would step in and take credit for CAL-PEP's hard work.

To gain the trust and support of staff, it became clear that CAL-PEP executive director, Gloria Lockett, should be named a coprincipal investigator. She assured the agency that this evaluation was in CAL-PEP's best interest and would not harm clients or the agency. Moreover, she saw the opportunity to satisfy funders and improve staff services. This project was what CAL-PEP needed.

It was then sociologist and researcher Benjamin Bowser's turn. He asked staff: "What are the things you have been curious about? What have you wanted to know about your clients and your work with them?" He told them he would help find answers to their questions, making the research useful to them. Initially, the staff challenged him, testing whether their views would be respected and taken to heart. Then they began to really answer his questions. Their main interest, they said, was not the evaluation of their work. They already knew plenty about clients' behavior—the risks they take that expose them to HIV infection. The high-risk behavior of drug addicts and sex workers, they said, gets studied over and over again.

Their question was deeper: Why do addicts and sex workers do what they do, putting themselves at repeated risk? They thought that if they knew why people become addicts and sex workers, they could devise better prevention. Little work has been done in the social and behavioral sciences to understand why people become addicts and sex workers. The staff hoped that researchers could provide insight.

Benjamin Bowser was asked "What are *your* hypotheses—what are you going to test?" To get them to outline their ideas and to get their cooperation, the researcher's theories and hypotheses had to be put on the table as well for staff to discuss and comment on.

Based on their experiences working with injection drug users and sex workers, the staff presented five core ideas they wanted to explore. Each of the five points was crafted into a research hypothesis:

1. A direct relationship occurs between injectors' and sex workers' marginal economic existence and their level of HIV risk taking. The greater and the longer their economic marginality, the higher their HIV risk.

2. A link exists between the age they started legitimate work and their risk of heavy drug use. Those who began heavy drug use after beginning their first full-time job seem to use more drugs, more often, compared to those who never worked or who began heavy drug use before their initial full-time job.

3. A connection exists between the level of a respondent's HIV high-risk behavior and his or her parents' knowledge of these risks. If parents know of their child's risks, the behaviors are either increased or decreased compared to those whose parents do not know.

4. Although sex workers continue to take HIV risks as a function of their "work," they and injectors have attempted to reduce risk through elaborate formulas that determine with whom they will, and will not, use condoms. There are many categories of sex partners: one-time paying clients, regular paying clients, main partners, regular nonpaying partners, and occasional nonpaying partners. Sex workers vary their condom use depending on the partners.

5. Many sex workers and drug-using clients have traded sex in jail. Did it make any difference in their HIV risk taking? Staff suspected that those who reported sex in jail might take greater risks on the streets.

None of these hypotheses appear in the research literature; all needed to be explored. The final idea is a point of curiosity that questions the usefulness and safety of some jails as sites for treatment and prevention.

The researcher had his own hypotheses. Bowser had to convince the staff of the importance of these ideas from the research literature.

They helped supplement these hypotheses with helpful contextual questions. He speculated that:

1. HIV risk behavior and sex trading are related to transgenerational (grandparents to parent to respondent) economic status. The lower the socioeconomic status (SES) of families, the greater their level of risk behaviors (Bluestone, 1983; Farley and Allen, 1989; Jaynes and Williams, 1989).
2. Restrictive and authoritarian family environments (based on the Moos family environment scale) are associated with injection drug use and sex trading (Moos, 1974, 1984).
3. Addicts, even as adults, are emotionally dependent upon their parents, according to M. Duncan Stanton's family theory of drug abuse. Unresolved deaths of close family members also may put someone at risk of adult drug abuse and HIV risk taking (Barth, Pietrak, and Ramier, 1993; Coleman, 1980; Mayer and Roberts, 1959; Stanton, 1980; Stanton and Todd, 1982).
4. The position one holds in family and friends' social networks influences the extent to which one injects drugs and engages in sex trading (Biegel, McCradle, and Mendelson, 1985; Bienenstock, Bonacich, and Oliver, 1990; Breiger, 1991; Friedman, 1995; Needle et al., 1995; Scott, 1991).
5. Injectors and sex workers who grow up in nuclear-organized families are more likely to take HIV risks than those who grow up in more extended organized families. This hypothesis is an extension of the work on black extended families (Shimkin and Uchendu, 1978; Stack, 1974; Sudarkasa, 1988).
6. A direct relationship occurs between the accumulation of early stressful life events, traumas, and later injection drug use and sex trading (Coleman, Kaplan, and Downing, 1986; Smith, 1992; Turner, Wheaton, and Lloyd, 1995).

The CAL-PEP staff encouraged researchers to explore more deeply the work and family backgrounds of clients and nonclients. As a result, the project was able to outline a much richer set of ideas for testing than if it had relied solely on the research literature or focused strictly on evaluation. By working with staff in defining the research questions, their support of the project was gained.

Once they were informed, supportive, and engaged in the evaluation, an important task in program evaluation had to be done. What staff actually did with clients in each program element had to be determined. Often, the ways in which program activities are described are different from what is actually done. Also, to interview clients about CAL-PEP services, the researchers had to understand how CAL-PEP provides services and learn the street terms used by clients. The research team had to understand what distinct groups of categorical services each street term referred to.

Provision of services is a complicated puzzle. Like all prevention programs, CAL-PEP relies on a variety of government and foundation funding sources. Since each funding source pays for specific services, CAL-PEP lists its programs according to these funding categories: education, health, and prevention (bleach for needles and condoms). For instance, health services are brought to clients from the county van and the "reach one teach one" educational efforts. The reality is that what the staff actually does with clients is very different from the program categories. The staff cannot deliver effective street services by working only within funding categories. They cannot address the funded needs of their clients and ignore needs that are not funded. Clients' needs and HIV risks are not neatly bound by funding categories.

For staff to be effective in keeping a relationship with clients and helping them reduce their HIV risk, they have to address clients' needs for housing, food, and money as well as their children's health, legal services, clothes, and safety. These needs are not directly funded through AIDS prevention dollars. Also, clients do not recognize the services they receive from CAL-PEP staff by their administrative categories. Service providers should be careful not to evaluate administrative categories that have no reality in the field. The actual services that the staff provides to clients *regardless* of funding categories should be evaluated.

For example, the "$25 drawing" was the clients' term for harm reduction workshops, because the staff uses a prize drawing to maximize attendance. "The chicken people" was a term given to CAL-PEP workers who give food away as an incentive to get people to participate in a safer-sex quiz, a condom demonstration, and role-playing on how to get partners to use condoms. "The condom people," "condom van," and "condom lady" were terms for the free condom and bleach distributions.

It became clear that clients might be coming to CAL-PEP services for more than money, referrals, food, and free condoms and bleach.

They might also visit because of positive relationships with staff. So several questions were added to the service evaluation section of the questionnaire to learn more about clients' relations with staff. The service evaluation form, in which clients were asked to identify and then rate each service, was then field tested with clients in pilot interviews. The quality of the questions, and the translation of administrative terms into familiar lingo, could not have been possible without full staff partnership in the research.

METHODS

Selecting Interview Staff

Interviewers

Collaboration did not stop with defining the research agenda and developing client-centered questions. What was learned from staff about their clients helped shape who was selected as interviewers and how interviews were selected.

For instance, it was concluded that only a small and selective number of injection drug users and sex workers would come to a "field site" such as a storefront office during the day for an interview. Rather, the best way to get a precise cross section of CAL-PEP clients and non-clients was to interview when and where CAL-PEP worked with clients. This meant interviewing on the streets, in crack houses, in shooting galleries, in single occupancy hotels at night, in the early morning—and doing follow-up interviews in jail.

Such interviews would require extraordinary interviewers who could handle themselves in street settings and be creative in finding private settings to conduct interviews. They had to establish rapport and trust with people who tend to be masters of manipulation. When paying subjects for their help, they had to handle money in dangerous settings. A team of inexperienced graduate students might be "eaten alive" or at least "conned." CAL-PEP prevention staff could not be used as interviewers due to the potential problem of bias.

The interviewer selection problem was also addressed through collaboration. Research and CAL-PEP principal investigators interviewed a pool of community people who were looking for work. With funding for four interviewers, two women and one man were selected who had experience on the streets and among injection drug users and sex workers. They were bright and articulate, could hold their own regardless of settings, and were excited about being trained as interviewers. The fourth interviewer was a graduate student with considerable street-based interviewing experience who served as team leader and cotrainer. It took six weeks to train the interview team and to conduct initial and pilot interviews.

Recruitment

Also addressed collaboratively was the challenge of selecting clients and nonclient injection drug users and sex workers for interviews. The goal was to compare CAL-PEP clients with nonclients to see if CAL-PEP services made a difference. Together, it was agreed to define CAL-PEP clients as sex workers and injection drug users who had utilized CAL-PEP services at least three times in the prior six months. Sex workers were self-identified and usually came to CAL-PEP services in small groups. Injection drug users also self-identified, were willing to show tracks, and were identified as users by other known injection drug users. All of the research subjects were actively engaged in sex trading and/or injection drug use.

Interviewers accompanied CAL-PEP outreach staff to their sites. At each site, a senior outreach worker was responsible for recruiting clients and nonclients for interviews. Male-female interview teams worked each site. Where there were numerous perspective interviewees, the outreach recruiter was asked to select every third client and nonclient they encountered. No one could be interviewed without first being selected by the outreach recruiter.

After determining eligibility, each perspective interviewee was introduced to an interviewer. The interviewer would review eligibility again to ensure that the subject was either an injection drug user and/or sex worker. If the person was not eligible, they were returned to the outreach worker. If they were eligible, the subject and interviewer would find a private place to conduct the interview.

Typical interview locations were fast-food shops, park benches, bus stop shelters, back stairs, inside subject and interviewer's cars, empty back rooms of houses and apartments, and empty street corners. Extensive locator information was collected from each person in order to re-recruit him or her one year later.

Conducting the Interviews

The project showed that collaborative research has both advantages and disadvantages. One major advantage was that the research was grounded in the mission of the organization. By working together, the teams did an excellent job in identifying, recruiting, and interviewing clients and nonclients. Because they conducted interviews where subjects lived, the team did not lose contact with clients. Clients who were recruited were interviewed on the spot, which allowed more accurate samples of clients and nonclients.

The fact that the interview team was street smart, could deal with "conning," could not be threatened, and was not averse to interviewing on the streets resulted with more authentic responses to questions. Moreover, the clients felt free to reveal sensitive information to the interviewers because of CAL-PEP's community base and years of work with them. CAL-PEP staff involvement paid off because outreach recruiters made a special effort to recruit for the evaluation project, in addition to doing their regular work. They also worked harder to observe the recruitment protocol and to find hard-to-find subjects than they would have in a field office. The recruiters had no problem finding nonclients. They were surprised to find how many sex workers and injection drug users had never used their services.

Since both research-based evaluators and CAL-PEP recruiters were in the field together, they were able to monitor and critique each other's work. Any problems in recruiting or interviewing were identified immediately and were dealt with. CAL-PEP staff quickly came to accept the interview teams as their peers, people who were able to work with injection drug users and sex workers on their turf, and accepted the evaluation project as important to the CAL-PEP mission. Interviewers acknowledged the skill and difficulty in working with street-based addicts and sex workers.

Another advantage of collaborative research became apparent when we had to find and reinterview the people we interviewed in the first year. One year after the initial interviews, 70 percent of first-year subjects were reinterviewed because of close rapport with outreach staff. Also, project staff was able to convince the interviewees' family members and friends of the importance of the interview in the second year. Despite the availability of "locator information" and the addresses and telephone numbers of people who knew them, it required extensive work on the part of CAL-PEP outreach staff to find many interviewees. Because interviewers had backgrounds on the streets, they were able to also do outreach to find clients and nonclients they had interviewed. When they finally found an interviewee, they conducted the interview on the spot.

Collaboration meant extra work, such as weekly team meetings with CAL-PEP staff. At these meetings we reviewed completed interviews, did scheduling, sought collective solutions to problems, resolved personal conflicts, reviewed and clarified procedure, planned for the coming week, and corrected questions in the questionnaire that were unclear or problematic. At these weekly meetings and during additional times, interviewers turned in completed questionnaires for review. Discrepancies were identified and resolved. Occasionally, the interview team would meet away from CAL-PEP, usually at the university, to reinforce their independence and identity apart from CAL-PEP. These off-site meetings were both retreats and training sessions. Several months into the project, interviewers were also trained to enter data from each other's questionnaires into Statistical Package for the Social Sciences Data Entry (SPSS/DE).

Not all of our experiences with collaborative research were positive. For instance, the university wished to identify perspective interviewers from its pool of people seeking employment, rather than from the more appropriate CAL-PEP pool of community people. The close working relation between evaluation staff and CAL-PEP staff led to conflict. One source of conflict was the fact that the interview staff's pay scale was higher than CAL-PEP staff, since the interviewers were employed and paid through the university. Because these two staffs worked closely together and were peers, they knew about their pay difference. Another source of conflict was CAL-PEP staff's out-of-pocket expenses for clients' food and other needs—expenses that were not covered by their funding. Since the interviewers were not engaged in prevention services, they had no out-of-pocket costs for clients.

The use of indigenous community talent as interviewers also had a price. Although these interviewers were excellent at interviewing sex workers and injection drug users, they had to acquire more professional attitudes as the project progressed. They did not start the project with professional attitudes; one particular challenge was learning to separate their personal lives from their work lives. As a result, there were more personal conflicts and interpersonal crises to resolve than one would have encountered with a more experienced and professional team. An additional problem occurred when one of the community interviewers was found to be forging interviews, and was fired. In the second year of the project, the more experienced and professional graduate student team leader had to be replaced on the project as well.

Overall, the cost in time and money involved in training new interviewers is higher than it is for an experienced team. Collaborative research requires more time to plan and to win nonresearch staff support. Because more voices and interests are involved, they all must be accommodated.

RESULTS AND COLLABORATIVE FINDINGS

Because of the research, CAL-PEP gained a better understanding of the clients and nonclients that were recruited and interviewed at the service sites in East and West Oakland. No significant differences occurred between the race, gender, and age of clients and nonclients (see Table 3.1). Clients had significantly higher incomes than nonclients. They used noninjection and injection drugs more often, had been infected with sexually transmitted diseases less often, were more likely to use crack cocaine, were less likely to have been to prison, and were more likely to have been in drug treatment at one time. These differences provide some sense of why injection-drug users and sex workers become CAL-PEP clients. However, sex workers and drug abusers have an additional purpose for which they use CAL-PEP. They come to CAL-PEP when their addiction and/or sex trading are spiraling out of control along with their HIV risks. Once they have regained control, they often stop using CAL-PEP services.

As a result, CAL-PEP clients are going to have, on average, higher rather than lower HIV risk levels. Only clients who make themselves available to all of the services over a period of time are going to successfully reduce their HIV risks. These are individuals who have the psychological and physical resources to go into treatment and to end

TABLE 3.1. CAL-PEP Clients and Nonclients: West and East Oakland Injectors and Sex Traders

	Client	Nonclient	p <
Race			
African American	130	168	0.771
White	4	10	
Hispanic	7	11	
Gender			
Female	102	121	0.228
Male	48	75	
Median age	41.3	39.4	0.073
Median income	$7,476	$5,831	0.025
	(N = 149)	(N – 205)	
Times inject drugs/month	42.2	29.7	0.022
	(N = 104)	(N = 124)	
Noninjection drugs used	2.3	1.9	0.028
	(N = 153)	(N = 207)	
Median STDs	2.08	3.35	0.012
	(N = 150)	(N = 196)	
Use crack?			
Yes	100	114	0.041
No	52	93	
Ever been to prison?			
Yes	38	80	0.006
No	111	123	
Drug treatment ever?			
Yes	77	78	0.013
No	74	128	

their sex trading and drug abuse. Because of this finding, CAL-PEP street-based services focus on harm reduction and HIV prevention rather than abstinence from drug use and sex trading. Although no one service component was found to reduce HIV risk alone, CAL-PEP services overall were important to clients in management of HIV risks.

In interviews with outreach staff, the reality of harm reduction and prevention as simultaneous goals becomes clear when observing how the staff works with clients. People come to CAL-PEP with their HIV risk-taking behavior embedded in their need to make money to support themselves, their families, and their addictions. They are isolated from opportunities to earn legitimate incomes because they have limited education, jail records, and inconsistent work backgrounds. So to address their HIV risk-taking behaviors, CAL-PEP staff must first address clients' need for housing, food, health care, legal problems, their children's needs, and security issues.

CAL-PEP is not funded to deal with such comprehensive needs. But through extensive referrals and force of personality, the staff tries to meet client needs. This is why the outreach staff sought to learn more about the circumstances and emotional histories of sex workers and injection drug use. They believe that once entering "the mix" of adversities, clients' lives are literally not their own. Sex trading and drug use take on a life of their own. The social context of CAL-PEP's outreach is important in any interpretation of the research data.

Staff-Based Findings

The success or failure of any research protocol is determined as follows: Were there insights? Can the hypotheses be demonstrated? To what extent can findings be generalized? Are the data high quality? It took time and effort to integrate staff insights about their clients into the research protocol. Was it worth it? Were their insights demonstrable? Table 3.2 reports the analysis of staff questions in the interviews.

The first staff hypothesis indicated a direct relationship between a client's ability to earn a living and HIV high-risk behavior. Clients and nonclients who believed work was important used, on average, fewer injection drugs ($p < .047$) and had fewer sexually transmitted diseases ($p < .004$) than those who thought work was not important. CAL-PEP staff believed those who thought work was important were more likely to seek employment—and, if they found a job, they were more likely to keep it. They concluded that a marginal work life and low participation in the economy reinforces more frequent drug use and greater HIV sexual risks. If this is true, then steady work in the legitimate economy is itself an HIV prevention measure.

TABLE 3.2. Staff-Based Findings

	Total	Mean	p <
	Number Injection Drugs Used Ever		
Steady work is important			
True	277	1.5	0.047
Somewhat true	42	1.6	
Somewhat false	5	2.6	
False	24	2.3	
	Number of STD Infections		
True	272	1.7	0.004
Somewhat true	41	3.7	
Somewhat false	5	4.0	
False	24	2.9	
	Number HIV Risk Categories		
When did you begin using drugs regularly?			
Before first job	177	3.55	0.045
After began work	118	3.0	
Never worked regularly	34	3.47	
	Number of STD Infections		
Before first job	178	2.27	0.009
After began work	118	1.33	
Never worked regularly	34	3.47	
	Number Injection Drugs Used Ever		
Before first job	57	2.82	0.048
After began work	141	2.41	
Never worked regularly	24	2.50	
	Number Injection Drugs Used/Thirty Days		
Parents know you use drugs			
Yes	257	1.10	0.042
No	72	0.68	

	Total	Mean	p <
		Frequency Sex with All Partners	
Parents know you use injection drugs			
Yes	142	5.77	0.026
No	71	9.32	
		Number HIV Risk Categories	
Sex in jail, ever			
Yes	38	4.55	0.000
No	320	3.21	
		Number STD Infections	
Yes	38	4.91	0.000
No	321	1.68	

The second staff hypothesis concerned work. Staff differed as to whether early work experience is associated with more or less drug use and sex trading over time. Several staff members believed that clients who started drugs after they began work use more drugs and sex trade more heavily than those who began their drug use before their first job or who never worked. Other staff members believed the opposite. Those who started drug use after their first job used fewer drugs and did less sex work. Table 3.2 shows the results across three measures of HIV risk taking—the number of HIV risks that one is engaged in, the number of STDs one has had, and the number of drugs one has injected. Those who began their drug use after their initial job showed consistently lower HIV risk levels when compared to those who began their drug use before their first job or who never worked. The basic insight here is that for adults some relationship exists between HIV risk taking and initial work experience. From hypothesis one and two, a positive attitude toward work and work experience prior to drug use and sex work appear to have a protective effect against HIV risks.

The third staff insight is that parental knowledge of drug use and sex risk can influence the risk of injection drug users and sex workers becoming HIV infected. The hypothesis is that parents' knowledge somehow results in lower HIV risk taking for their adult child. Here the results in Table 3.2 are conflicting. Respondents who reported that their parents knew that they were injection drug users used on average more drugs in the month prior to the interview than those who reported that their parents did not know (1.10 drugs versus 0.68 drugs, p < .042). The results were just the opposite for the frequency of sex with all partners in the prior month. Respondents whose parents knew of their HIV risk behavior had sex fewer times (5.77) than those whose parents did not know (9.32 times). We do not know enough about this issue to answer the question of why parents' knowledge has opposite effects for drug and sex risks. The hypothesis itself may be problematic. Whichever the case, staff have identified a new statistically significant factor that appears to impact HIV risk taking (p < .026) that is well worth exploring.

The fourth staff hypothesis was that injection drug users and sex workers use condoms selectively, depending upon whether or not they are having sex with their main, regular, or casual partners. We found no statistically significant relationships between condom use with type of partners and HIV high-risk behaviors.

Finally, the staff explored whether an experience of sex in jail made any difference in high HIV risk. Among respondents, 10.6 percent (N = 38) claimed that they had sex in jail. These individuals were currently engaged in more HIV risks (p < .000) and had more lifetime STDs (p < .000) than those who did not report having sex in jail. This finding suggests that we need to know much more about what goes on in jail, such as rape, men having sex with men, sex for money or survival, and drug use. Also it should not be automatically assumed that jail is a safe and HIV risk-free setting. Therefore, it is an appropriate place for HIV prevention, and drug treatment and prevention.

Researcher-Based Findings

Tables 3.3 and 3.4 report analysis of the researcher-based questions in the interviews. There were several significant relationships between father and grandparent's social economic status, and four HIV high-risk behaviors. In Table 3.3, all of the injection-drug users and sex workers interviewed are considered in the lower socioeconomic class because of their limited educational attainment, low income, and work history. Based upon reports of their mothers', fa-

TABLE 3.3. Researcher-Based Findings

	Total	Mean	p <
	Number Injection Drugs Ever Used		
Father's SES			
Low	39	1.84	0.000
Working	206	1.83	
Middle	19	1.78	
Don't Know	79	0.89	
	Number Injection Drugs Used in Thirty Days		
Low	39	1.20	0.011
Working	206	1.15	
Middle	19	0.79	
Don't Know	79	0.51	
	Number Noninjecction Drugs Used Three+/Week		
Grandparent's SES			
Low	34	3.20	0.026
Working	90	2.95	
Middle	20	3.10	
Don't Know	200	2.33	
	Number Injection Drugs Used Last Thirty Days		
Low	34	1.79	0.011
Working	90	1.00	
Middle	20	1.05	
Don't Know	200	0.84	

thers', and grandfathers' occupations, an approximation was made regarding their parents' socioeconomic status (SES). The lower a respondent father's SES, the higher on average were the number of injection drugs ever used ($p < .000$) and the number of injection drugs used thirty days prior to the interview ($p < .011$).

A puzzling finding in this analysis is that respondents who did not know what their father's occupation was had the lowest rates of drug use. This is puzzling because the assumption was made that those with the least knowledge of their family and history would have higher drug abuse.

TABLE 3.4. Researcher-Based Findings (Correlation Coefficient/p < /N)

	Types sex partners	Noninject drugs ever	Noninject Drugs 3+/wk	Inject drugs ever	Inject drugs 30 days	Number STDs	Exchange partner 30 days	Number HIV Risks
Moos family environment			0.120 / 0.025 / 345	0.110 / 0.040 / 345	-0.115 / 0.033 / 345		0.129 / 0.017 / 338	
Number deaths		0.141 / 0.008 / 348	0.262 / 0.000 / 348				-0.183 / 0.000 / 341	
Closeness with family	0.215 / 0.000 / 341				-0.111 / 0.038 / 347			
Extended family		-0.154 / 0.004 / 339	-0.143 / 0.008 / 339	-0.127 / 0.019 / 339		-0.112 / 0.040 / 333		-0.132 / 0.015 / 340

Life event/12 months	0.115	0.189	0.193	0.253		0.138	0.145	0.183
	0.033	0.000	0.000	0.000		0.011	0.007	0.001
	341	347	347	347		341	340	340
Current chronic stress	0.289		0.126	0.160				0.122
	0.000		0.019	0.003				0.024
	341		347	347				340
Childhood traumas		0.149	0.181	0.204	0.241	0.182		
		0.005	0.001	0.000	0.000	0.001		
		347	347	347	347	341		
Lifetime traumas		0.267	0.286	0.167	0.360			
		0.000	0.000	0.002	0.000			
		347	347	347	347			

The same general pattern was evident in respondents' HIV risks related to grandfathers' SES. The lower the grandfather's SES, the more often three or more noninjection drugs were used in the week prior to the interview (p < .026) and the greater the number of injection drugs used in the past thirty days (p < .011). Respondents with working-class grandfathers or who did not know their grandfathers' occupations had slightly lower drug abuse rates. This is the first time intergenerational SES has been used and found significantly related to HIV risk levels.

Table 3.4 shows the findings for the other hypotheses. The Moos Family Environment scale measured the extent to which one experienced a restrictive family environment in which self-expression was discouraged and even punished. Scale measures were significantly correlated to four HIV risk measures. The more restrictive the environment during a client's formative years, the more noninjection drugs they used per week (p < .025), the more likely they injected (p < .040), and the more sex exchanges they engaged in the month before their interview (p < .017). Higher-than-average sudden deaths of close family members in the years prior to injecting or sex work also were found to be significantly related to three HIV risk measures (number of noninjection drugs ever used (p < .008), the number of noninjection drugs used three or more times per week (p < .000), and the numbers of sex exchange partners (p < .000). Drug abuse was connected to the loss of close family members by the emotional ties between the addict and their parents (close relations). This closeness reinforces through family dynamics their identity as drug abusers.

In a measure of respondents' interactions with family—degree of closeness—the greater the family closeness and contact, the greater the number of respondents' sex partners (p <.000). All of the correlations between extended family organization and HIV high risk were negative. Respondents with family organizations that were more nuclear rather than more extended were more likely to engage in risky HIV behaviors. Families organized around grandparents, aunts, and uncles were less likely to result in HIV high-risk behaviors. Respondents from the more culturally accepted nuclear families were more apt to be HIV high-risk takers.

Four social stress measures (multiple crises in past twelve months, chronic stress, childhood trauma, lifetime trauma) were positively related to HIV risk taking. People with accumulated life events (burned out of housing, sudden death of close relatives, arrest, loss of job, illness) in the year prior to their interview reported higher HIV risk taking. Those with higher numbers of specific chronic stress, childhood traumas, and lifetime traumas all reported higher HIV risk taking than those with lower or little stress and trauma.

CONCLUSION

This research project began with two goals: (1) improve science, and (2) yield findings useful for HIV prevention. The science should be community-based so that the scientific hypotheses could be tested as close as possible to the people who engage in HIV high-risk behavior. Prevention science is not field site research, where science is done somewhere in downtown offices and the community is simply a field site to test the scientific ideas. Community-based work creates the opportunity to gain a better sense of the context of how and why people risk their lives against a disease such as AIDS. One can learn, not simply what high-risk takers do, but why they do it—in other words, the social context of risk takers' behavior.

With these goals in mind, this project began with several key assumptions about what collaborative research should entail. First, CAL-PEP was to be a full partner in defining and conducting the research. Second, the staff has insights and knowledge about their clients based on years of experience working with drug abusers and sex workers. Some staff members were once clients themselves and had been HIV high-risk takers.

The results of this research—both the process and its findings—affirmed initial goals. The science was improved. Its results are potentially useful to CAL-PEP in improving its prevention efforts. Furthermore, the experience and results were not unique; other science and prevention teams can replicate this collaborative research experience. Although this chapter focused primarily on the new research findings, the evaluation also benefited from the project's collaborative method.

CAL-PEP is working toward change. Drug abusers and sex workers come to CAL-PEP street outreach teams with complex interrelated problems, of which only one is HIV risk. Staff could not address the HIV risk without also addressing the other problems. Clients need housing, food, and medical attention. They have legal problems, children to care for, and their lives are in continuous crisis. Most are cut off from the legitimate economy due to their drug abuse and criminal records. Many have multiple traumas and psychological problems that are unaddressed. But most important, these people earn their living through sex trading and selling drugs. They are locked into taking risks that are literally structured into their lives. To reduce their HIV risk without extensive supportive services means not simply reducing their addictions, drug abuse, and sex trading—it also means reducing their incomes and ability to survive day-to-day. Yet CAL-PEP is funded only to address their HIV risk taking.

Given clients' realities, it is no coincidence that no single CAL-PEP HIV prevention measure significantly reduced clients' HIV risk taking. But overall, CAL-PEP services were found to have a positive effect. Despite barriers to HIV prevention, drug abusers and sex workers who took advantage of CAL-PEP services were able to stabilize their drug use and reduce some of their HIV risks.

People whose drug abuse and sex trading are spiraling out of control, boosting their HIV risks, come to CAL-PEP. CAL-PEP's mission in the mainstream world of funders, the press, and federal government is to prevent HIV infection. However, that mission among drug abusers and sex workers is different. For them, CAL-PEP is their bridge to comprehensive services that are one-stop and full service. They use CAL-PEP to reduce their harm and lower their likelihood of getting HIV infection. Yet they will continue to take HIV risks as long as they are injectors and sex workers.

Finally, this collaborative research model is not complete; it did not include the insights of clients in the research. Injectors and sex workers, who would offer an additional rich source of insight, were not included in definitions of the research questions. Much more needs to be learned and tested.

REFERENCES

Ashery, R. S., Carlson, R. G., Falck, R. S., and Siegal, H. A. (1995). Injection drug users, crack-cocaine users, and human services utilization: An exploratory study. *Social Work, 40*(1), 75-82.

Astemborski, J., Vlahov, D., Warren, D., Solomon, L., and Nelson, K. E. (1994). The trading of sex for drugs or money and HIV seropositivity among female intravenous drug users. *American Journal of Public Health, 84*(3), 382-387.

Barth, R. P., Pietrak, J., and Ramier, M. (Ed.) (1993). *Families Living with Drugs and HIV: Intervention and Treatment Strategies.* New York: Guilford Press.

Biegel, D. E., McCradle, E., and Mendelson, S. (1985). *Social Networks and Mental Health: An Annotated Bibliography.* Beverly Hills: Sage Publications.

Bienenstock, E. J., Bonacich, P., and Oliver, M. (1990). The effect of network density and homogeneity on attitude solarization. *Social Networks, 12,* 153-172.

Bluestone, B. (1983). Deindustrialization and unemployment in America. *Review of Black Political Economy, 12*(3), 27-42.

Breiger, R. L. (1991). *Explorations in Structural Analysis: Dual and Multiple Networks of Social Interaction.* New York: Garland.

Coleman, S. (1980). Incomplete mourning and addiction: Family transactions. In D. J. Lettieri, Sayers, M., and Pearson, H.W. (Eds.), *Theories of Drug Abuse,* Volume 30 (pp. 83-89). Washington, DC: NIDA.

Coleman, S. B., Kaplan J. D., and Downing, R. W. (1986). Life cycle and loss—the spiritual vacuum of heroin addiction. *Family Process, 25,* 5-23.

Farley, R. and Allen, W. R. (Eds.) (1989). *The Color Line and the Quality of Life in America.* New York: Oxford University Press.

Friedman, S. R. (1995). Summary: Promising social network research results and suggestions for a research agenda. In S. R. Friedman (Ed.), *Social Networks, Drug Abuse and HIV Transmission,* Volume 151 (pp. 196-215). Bethesda: NIDA Monograph.

Jaynes, G. D. and Williams Jr., R. M. (Eds.) (1989). *Common Destiny: Blacks and American Society.* Washington, DC: National Academy Press.

Mayer, J. K. and Roberts, B.H. (1959). *Family and Class Dynamics in Mental Illness.* New York: Wiley.

Moos, R. (1974). *Evaluating Treatment Environments: A Social Ecological Approach.* New York: Wiley-Interscience.

Moos, R. (1984). *The Family Environment Scale.* Palo Alto, CA: Counseling Psychology Press.

Needle, R., Coyle, S., Genser, S. G., and Trotter, R. T. (Eds.) (1995). *Social Networks, Drug Abuse, and HIV Transmission* (Volume 151). Rockville, MD: NIDA.

Reardon, J. (1994). *HIV/AIDS Epidemiology Profile of the East Bay, California (Alameda and Contra Costa Counties).* Oakland, CA: Alameda County Health Care Services Agency.

Scott, J. (1991). *Social Network Analysis: A Handbook.* Newbury Park, CA: Sage.

Shimkin, D. B. and Uchendu, V. (1978). Persistence, borrowing, and adaptive changes in black kinship systems: Some issues and their significance. In D. Shimkin, Shimkin, E., and Frate, D.A. (Eds.), *The Extended Family in Black Societies* (pp. 391-406). The Hague: Mouton Publishers.

Smith, T. (1992). A life events approach to developing an index of societal well-being. *Social Science Research, 21,* 353-379.

Stack, C. (1974). *All Our Kin.* New York: Harper.

Stanton, M. D. (1980). A family theory of drug abuse. In Lettieri D.J., Sayers, M., and Pearson, H.W. (Eds.), *Theories on Drug Abuse,* Volume 30 (pp. 147-156). Washington, DC: NIDA.

Stanton, M. D. and Todd, T. C. (1982). *The Family Therapy of Drug Abuse and Addiction.* New York: Guilford Press.

Sudarkasa, N. (1988). Interpreting the African heritage in Afro-American family organization. In H. P. McAdoo (Ed.), *Black Families* (pp. 27-43). Thousand Oaks, CA: Sage.

Turner, J., Wheaton, B., and Lloyd, D. A. (1995). The epidemiology of social stress. *American Sociological Review, 60,* 104-125.

Watters, J. K., Bluthental, R. N., and Kral, A. H. (1995). HIV seroprevalence in injection drug users (letter). *Journal of the American Medical Association, 273,* 15, 1178.

Chapter 4

Collaborative Research Toward HIV Prevention Among Migrant Farmworkers

Shiraz I. Mishra
Fernando Sanudo
Ross F. Conner

As the HIV crisis has grown, many prevention programs have been developed to stop the spread of HIV. However, few if any of these programs have addressed the specific unmet HIV prevention needs of migrant farmworkers. Moreover, except for one study (Mishra, Connor, and Magaña, 1996; Mishra and Conner, 1996), there has been no body of research that addresses HIV prevention education among farmworkers.

Migrant farmworkers are in dire need of prevention information due to risk factors such as unsafe sexual practices, use of injection drugs, and unsanitary living conditions. They are among the most challenging of populations to reach due to their migrant status and social and linguistic isolation.

Although the majority of male Latino farmworkers are married, they often live without their families at farm camps (Mishra, Conner, and Magaña, 1996; Mishra and Conner, 1996). Sex workers regularly visit farmworkers, providing quick and inexpensive services for the men in the fields. It is not uncommon to see farmworkers queue up to purchase sex from a single sex worker, visiting the camps on payday to offer her services behind trees, in bushes, and in make-shift rooms—without proper sanitation facilities or any opportunity to clean herself between clients. Farmworkers also resist using condoms and are willing to pay sex workers extra money just to enjoy sex without a condom.

Vista Community Clinic, an AIDS Service Organization (ASO), based in north San Diego County has been in the forefront of HIV prevention efforts among low-income, hard-to-reach, and high-risk populations such as farmworkers and sex workers. Their efforts have included prevention education outreach activities such as distribution of informational materials, presentations and distribution of condoms, HIV testing and counseling, and provision of on-site medical care. However, the ASO had not conducted a rigorous scientific evaluation of its education outreach activities.

In this chapter, we describe a collaborative effort between the ASO and the University of California-Irvine (UC Irvine) to save the lives of migrant farmworkers and their families through safe sex education. We outline the challenges faced by collaborating university- and community-based institutions in the development, implementation, and evaluation of two innovative HIV prevention education programs that targeted migrant farmworkers. Finally, we describe the successes and failures of our mission in an effort to guide those undertaking similar collaborative projects.

THE COLLABORATION

Prior to initiation of the collaboration, the ASO's outreach staff had observed that farmworkers engaged in behaviors that placed them at a higher risk for HIV. Disturbingly, the ASO's clinical staff regularly treated a disproportionate number of farmworkers for sexually transmitted diseases. The ASO realized that community outreach alone, without a well-tailored education program, was unsuccessful in reducing the risk and incidence of HIV among farmworkers.

The ASO was approached in 1991 by UC-Irvine academicians seeking to collaborate on a research project that targeted Latino farmworkers. The ASO viewed this inquiry as an opportunity to not only research this population, but also to provide it with a much-needed service centered around HIV prevention education.

The two institutions collaborated on a pilot evaluation of HIV education and prevention materials (*Tres Hombres sin Fronteras* [Three Men without Borders] and *Marco Aprende como Protegerse* [Marco Learns How to Protect Himself]). The pilot evaluation indicated that the educational materials could be an effective tool to address the unmet HIV prevention needs of Spanish-speaking farmworkers with low literacy levels. More important, the pilot study provided invaluable insights into the conduct of collaborative research at the community level among a marginalized, hard-to-reach population (Mishra and Conner, 1996).

We followed this collaborative effort with a series of smaller collaborative studies that addressed HIV prevention policies and programmatic implications at the local, state, and national levels (Conner, Mishra, and Magaña, 1996; Conner, Mishra, and Magaña, 1998). These studies integrated research-based recommendations on HIV prevention with farmworkers' concerns about the utility of the researchers' recommendations. Moreover, we conducted feasibility assessments of the researchers' recommendations using state- and federal-level policymakers and administrators involved in HIV and AIDS policies and programs.

Until this point, the collaboration between the ASO and UC Irvine was limited in scope. The researchers would conceptualize the issues, design the study, obtain the funding, and analyze and report the data. The ASO provided access to the study population, helped implement the project in the field, offered outreach workers to conduct interviews, and solicited feedback from the community on interpretation of some of the findings. But the ASO and UC Irvine worked together only on implementation and interpretation of the projects. Although our prior collaborations were predominantly "university-controlled," they helped the collaborative partners understand and appreciate their respective expertise, institutional work cultures and capabilities, and community-based networks. Both the community and academic partners felt that this initial "controlled" phase of our collaborative efforts had positive ramifications for long-term collaborative efforts. Up to that point, the university controlled everything, so the ASO sometimes felt exploited. As a result of this collaboration, the ASO had the opportunity to participate more fully and learn more about research.

These efforts helped build an association between the two institutions, and more important, between the two primary institutional representatives, based on mutual trust, respect, and transparency; thus, setting the stage for a "true" collaborative effort. The University-wide AIDS Research Program (UARP) Collaborative AIDS Prevention Initiative provided an ideal framework to test the maturation of the collaboration between Vista Community Clinic and UC Irvine.

A Case History

True to the letter and spirit of the UARP initiative, the project began with a series of meetings between the university and ASO PIs and the ASO's community outreach staff. During these meetings, we had frank discussions about all aspects of the project—from grant writing responsibilities to scientific methodology. For the most part, these meetings were extremely cordial and frank, with everyone eager to express their views and ideas. Needless to say, we had moments when the challenges of the science and service dichotomy posed what seemed at times intractable differences. Given the importance of the issues under consideration, one of the truisms to emerge from our meetings was the art of compromise!

The goal of the collaboration was to change behavior among migrant farmworkers, inducing them to routinely use condoms during sex with a sex worker. We sought to measure whether ASO's outreach efforts in HIV prevention among low-literacy, male, Spanish-speaking, migrant farmworkers were effective in changing knowledge and behavior.

THE STUDY

Identifying the Target Population

The ASO's HIV prevention outreach efforts target many populations including farmworkers (migrant and seasonal), nursery workers, sex workers, and low-income Latino families. Preliminary research and seroprevalence studies of farmworkers corroborate some of the anecdotal accounts by outreach workers of sex practices that put farmworkers at risk of acquiring HIV when they arrive in the United States. One farmworker said: "They are different here, I met *gabachas* (North American women) that enjoy doing it in different ways. In Mexico, I only knew how to do it from the front and I never had oral sex with a girl, but I do it over here and I like them to do it to me. I learned better ways to do it: on my knees, mutual oral, she on top, standing up and sometimes anal" (Bronfman and Moreno, 1996).

Sex between men also occurs, although cultural proscriptions against same-sex behavior inhibit them from discussing the practice. A farmworker recounted his sexual experiences: "[A]bout everything, I masturbate them, suck them and they penetrate me, they like me to play the role of a woman" (Bronfman and Moreno, 1996). For some farmworkers, sex with other men is a way for them to stay faithful to their wives. As one farmworker noted:

> I cannot do strange things with my wife, she only does the regular things. She is a Protestant and I respect her, because I love her. But sometimes I would like to do things; many times I go all the way to Seaside to watch sex videos. When I go to the videos there is always someone who wants to suck you, and one gets hot, and sometimes I allow them to suck me. (Bronfman and Moreno, 1996)

Condom use among Latino farmworkers is reportedly very low, thus exposing them to infection. This is especially true for immigrant farmworkers who are more likely to report never having used a condom. Reasons for nonuse include a lack of sensitivity, discomfort of the partner, fear that it will be left "inside."

Farmworkers' isolated and substandard living conditions add to their HIV risk, making them more susceptible to disease. Farmworkers generally find themselves isolated, not only because of limited housing and mobility but also because of language difficulties. Camps range from holes in the ground (called spider holes) to enclosures made of old mattresses or cardboard pieces. In some cases, the camps are rooms with several bunk beds. Generally, there is poor nutrition, no sanitation, and inadequate safe drinking water in the camps (Mishra, Conner, and Magaña, 1996).

In view of these realities, coupled with the fact that the ASO wanted to assess the impact of its education programs for farmworkers, we decided that our HIV prevention efforts would be most effective if we targeted low-literacy, male, Spanish-speaking, migrant farmworkers.

We chose this population fully realizing that language and legal barriers posed serious challenges toward the development, implementation, evaluation, and institutionalization of effective culturally sensitive and linguistically appropriate HIV prevention programs. Although we were extremely interested in including sex workers in the program, budgetary constraints and sample-size issues precluded us from evaluating an educational program among them. We did, however, include sex workers in our study design and collected baseline information on their sexual practices.

Defining the Research Questions

The ASO has provided education and distributed condoms to migrant farmworkers since 1987. The education programs have ranged from simply distributing informative materials to didactic, classroom-style education sessions. However, evaluation of the programs was limited to a simple pretest and posttest survey on knowledge-based items. Moreover, when the farmworkers were asked how many had used a condom before the education and how many intended to use a condom after the education, nearly all the participants would raise their hands in response to both questions. (Apparently, the designated group "boss" would cue the desired behavior!)

As a consequence, the ASO had no evidence about the effectiveness of its programs. Moreover, in addition to an assessment of program effectiveness, the ASO wanted a scientific inquiry on how best to transfer information that was both culturally sensitive and resulted in positive behavior changes that did not regress over time. Specifically, the ASO was interested to know which method of education was more effective over time, simply distributing educational materials or providing an in-depth discussion about the educational materials. The ASO also hoped to understand why some men changed their behaviors and others did not. Last, both the community and academic partners felt that much of the gains of conducting HIV education in isolation (i.e., without incorporating the hierarchy of needs of the farmworkers such as jobs, housing, food) may be short-lived.

The scientific literature has numerous examples of effective programs for different populations, however, none of the work referred to the unique circumstances that surround migrant farmworkers.

With this in mind, we formulated the following research questions.

1. Do the ASO's outreach efforts change knowledge and behavior?
2. Which approach to education (distributing materials or holding discussions about materials) is most effective in changing knowledge and behavior?
3. What are the social, normative, and cultural factors that facilitate or impede behavior change?

Based on these research questions, we postulated the following hypotheses. At the posttest, farmworkers exposed to the education programs ("intervention") compared with those not exposed will:

1. have higher levels of HIV-related knowledge;
2. be more likely to report behavior change, that is, condom use during sex with a sex worker; and
3. be more likely to display adeptness (mastery) in behavioral skills such as use of condoms and initiation of interactions regarding protective practices.

At the posttest, farmworkers who received a greater "dose" of the intervention (i.e., exposed to discussions centered around the materials) compared with those who received only the materials will:

4. be more likely to report behavior change due to positive group dynamics, that is, due to interactions occurring within their group that are conducive for behavior change; and,
5. report greater positive changes, with behavior changes observed on long-term change analysis.

Study Design

We used a complex scientific design that helped us measure both short- and long-term changes in knowledge and behaviors, testing two versions of the educational program. The design included both quantitative (survey research) and qualitative (focus group) research methodologies. Figure 4.1 provides a schematic representation of the study design. In brief, we conducted the study in farmworker campsites, which we randomly assigned to three groups, two experimental groups (i.e., groups that received a version of the educational program) and a control group (which received the educational program at the end of the study). We followed eligible farmworkers in these groups over a period of about five months. During this period we administered a baseline survey (pretest) and two posttest surveys, and conducted focus groups with farmworkers who changed their behaviors (i.e., used a condom during sex with a sex worker) and those who did not change their behaviors. Farmworkers in the two experimental

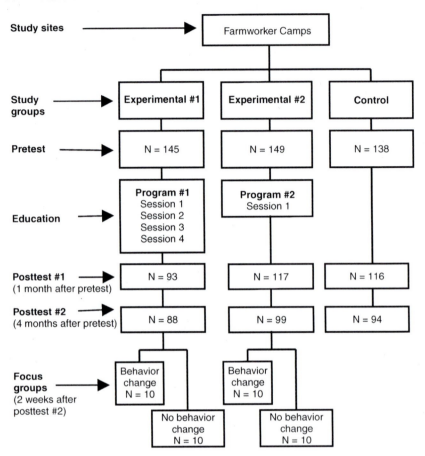

FIGURE 4.1. Program Implementation and Evaluation Design

groups received the respective versions of the educational program after the pretest survey.

The HIV Prevention Education

The first version of the educational program (Program #1) consisted of facilitated group discussions which, besides discussing HIV, encouraged the farmworkers to incorporate their social realities such as concerns about their families, jobs, money, and meals into the discussions. Program #1 took an interactive approach, allowing farmworkers to discuss in a group setting all of their concerns, such as living conditions, food, and medical care—not just HIV. The second version (Program #2) consisted of simply distributing the materials to the farmworkers, an activity that was part of the ASO's ongoing HIV prevention outreach efforts.

The educational materials included the *Tres Hombres sin Fronteras* [Three Men without Borders] *fotonovela* [a photo story book] and a *radionovela* [a radio story], and the *Marco Aprende como Protegerse* [Marco Learns How to Protect Himself] *fotonovela*.[1] The primary focus of the materials was to educate the farmworkers about HIV prevention. Condom use during sex with a sex worker was the prevention method given primary consideration. Behaviors such as needle sharing and sexual abstinence were noted in the program but were not a major focus.

Mapping the Study Sites

We conducted the study in North San Diego county, the geographical area served by the ASO. We mapped twenty-seven farmworker campsites within this region. These sites were clustered within a thirty-mile radius west, north, and southeast of the ASO. We randomly assigned these sites to the two experimental groups and the control group.

During the planning phase of the project, the research team (academic and community principal investigators and outreach workers) visited several farmworker campsites. The purpose of these visits was to apprise the academic partner of the logistic challenges for the fieldwork and living conditions within the campsites. In addition, these visits provided the academic partner the opportunity to directly interact with farmworkers, inquire about their needs, and to witness the social dynamics of sex workers soliciting farmworkers near the agricultural fields.

Initially, the farmworkers were hesitant to accept the academic partner into the campsites and viewed him with suspicion. However, after some initial resistance, the excellent rapport between the outreach workers and the camp residents helped break the ice and the academic partner was viewed as nonthreatening.

Outreach workers were also initially hesitant. Although the academic and community PIs had known each other and worked together for several years and shared mutual respect and trust, the outreach workers were less forthcoming in their acceptance of the academic PI. Behind the outward appearance of the culturally appropriate respect and professionalism, there was always an undercurrent of misgiving, mistrust, hesitancy, and reluctance directed toward the academic PI. It was an attitude that signaled: "We know what we are doing and do not need an outsider to tell us what to do, how to do it, and who to study."

It was only after the outreach workers saw the academic PI try to reach out to the farmworkers and share their concerns and experiences that they began accepting him as an equal. This was one of the many important transitions in our collaborative relationship as it signaled that finally the whole research team was working toward a common goal.

Recruitment of Farmworkers

The ASO's excellent rapport in the community greatly facilitated our entry into the farmworker campsites. The ASO informed all the farm owners about the study and we received unqualified support from the majority of them. The ASO also informed the Immigration and Naturalization Service (INS) and the local police department about our work with the farmworkers and sex workers. Without the ASO's credibility and community support, we may not have been in a position to achieve our desired goals. A description of the recruitment criteria and sample size of farmworkers is provided in the Appendix.

Despite the community support, however, we lost 151 farmworkers to attrition due to factors that we believe were not related to the study. First, some farmworkers recruited into the study lost their jobs and had to move to other parts of the state in search of employment. Second, a few farmworkers felt we were favoring some of them over others. Third, several campsites were faced with forced evictions and demolitions to make way for formal housing developments. Fourth, union activists attempting to organize the campsites misrepresented our work, linking us to "big business" interests or the law enforcement authorities. Fifth, the INS conducted raids in campsites believed to house farmworkers without proper U.S. work authorization permits. Last, a few of the farm owners and their supervisors believed that we would undermine their absolute control over the lives and working conditions of farmworkers by empowering them with knowledge and services. For a time, an atmosphere of open hostility occurred between our outreach workers and some farm owners and the relationship with the farmworkers was suspiciously nervous.

In the midst of this volatile environment, an unfortunate incident nearly cost the life of one of our outreach workers. Unbeknown to us, one of the campsites in our study was the target of an impending INS raid. On the appointed day, one of our outreach workers unsuspectingly entered the campsite and began collecting the farmworkers for their interviews. The camp supervisor, noticing the outreach worker's activity, ordered him to leave the campsite. The outreach worker tried to calm the supervisor and plead the case of the farmworkers, only to be verbally and physically abused. When the outreach worker stood his ground, the supervisor pulled out a handgun and threatened the life of the outreach worker. The outreach worker left the campsite, sending word to all the eligible farmworkers to meet him outside the campsite gate for their scheduled interview. We completed some interviews at the campsite, but achieved a much smaller number than we had initially recruited.

Measures

We constructed the surveys based on our prior work and with feedback from the outreach workers. The outreach workers were instrumental in ensuring that the length and content of the instrument was appropriate for the target population. They helped ensure that sufficient time was provided to conduct the surveys at the campsites after the farmworkers returned from their work but before it got dark. In addition, the outreach workers helped carefully word the questions so that low-literacy Spanish-speaking workers from rural backgrounds could understand and answer them accurately.

The surveys included questions on sociodemographics; HIV-related knowledge and practices; behavioral risk factors; personal experiences with HIV; and health care access. Extent of exposure, comprehension, and cultural sensitivity of the intervention was measured at posttest #1. Sociodemographic variables included age, marital status, education level, acculturation level, and ability to speak Spanish.

Acculturation level was based on the preferred language (Spanish or English) used to read, speak, think, talk with friends, and when growing up (Marin, Otero-Sabogal, and Perez-Stable, 1987). Twenty-six items measured knowledge about HIV transmission, treatment, and prognosis. Since the practice of primary interest was condom use, farmworkers were questioned as to whether they had had sex (ever and in the past one month) with their wife, girlfriend, sex worker, and another man—and whether they had used a condom in these instances.

Data Collection Procedures

The outreach workers were specially trained to conduct the surveys (see Figure 4.1 for implementation schedule). The surveys averaged about one hour and were conducted at the campsites. Outreach workers conducted the surveys in small groups (of about ten farmworkers per group), using a combination of survey administration techniques which have proved very successful in eliciting responses from participants who cannot read but can comprehend the spoken word and match icons in selecting responses. After the posttest #2 survey, the outreach workers conducted the focus groups. Two specially trained outreach workers administered the educational programs. The Human Subjects Review Committee of the University of California, Irvine, approved the research protocols for the surveys and educational program. We obtained written informed consent from all participants (which was read to them).

Educational Program Implementation Procedures

Program #1, implemented for experimental group #1, consisted of the two *fotonovelas,* two *radionovela,* and group discussions on topics contained in the educational materials. The outreach workers conducted four group discussion sessions each lasting about two hours and held twice per week for two weeks. During the sessions, the outreach workers posed questions to the participants that were designed to encourage discussion about HIV risk factors, prevention, and treatment of the disease and the potential impact of HIV infection on their lives. The outreach workers then guided the group to come up with solutions to the problem of the HIV epidemic as it affected members of the group.

The first module focused on HIV-related knowledge and myths and facts regarding the disease, with the men assessing how much they knew about HIV. The second module focused on learning about risk factors, symptoms, and the severity of HIV. The men set personal goals for behavior, a step designed to elevate their own expectations of themselves. The third module addressed prevention methods such as condom and needle use. The fourth module focused on issues of testing and personal risk assessment, concluding with a review of all material.

Program #2, implemented for experimental group #2, consisted of the two *fotonovelas* and broadcast of the *radionovela* during one two-hour meeting. Materials were not discussed during the session, although we do not rule out the possibility of some discussion occurring among the participants. Unlike in Program #1, the outreach workers did not link information to specific skills.

Farmworkers in the control group received the *fotonovelas* after completion of the posttest #2 surveys. All eligible farmworkers in the two experimental groups received the full complement of their respective educational program.

RESEARCH FINDINGS

Farmworker Characteristics

In the selection and randomization of farmworkers, our goal was to create comparable study groups. To verify that this had occurred, we compared a few sociodemographic characteristics between the two experimental groups and the control group and found no significant differences. The majority of farmworkers in the study were aged eighteen to twenty-five years, currently single, with less than seven years of education, little acculturation into American society, and literate in Spanish only.

We also compared selected sociodemographic characteristics of farmworkers in the study with those who left the study after the pretest. With one exception, no significant differences occurred between these farmworkers on indicators such as marital status, level of education, acculturation level, and ability to read Spanish. Proportionally more farmworkers in the study were aged eighteen to twenty-five years (65 percent versus 55 percent, p = .05).

HIV Knowledge

The educational programs significantly enhanced knowledge among farmworkers. The gain in knowledge was much lower among farmworkers in experimental group #2 than group #1. Figure 4.2 presents the median knowledge index scores for the three study groups at the pretest, posttest #1, and posttest #2. At the pretest, a high prevalence of misconceptions occurred regarding HIV. These misconceptions were reflected on the median scores of the knowledge index, which ranged from thirteen (control group) to fourteen (experimental groups #1 and #2). These scores indicated that about one-half of the farmworkers correctly identified only about one-half of the knowledge items.

We also conducted analysis of covariance to examine whether the impact of the two educational programs on knowledge scores was statistically significant. We modeled the analyses to uncover, after controlling for pretest (or posttest #1) scores, main effects of the two educational programs on posteducation (posttest #1 or posttest #2) knowledge scores. At posttest #1, controlling for pretest scores, farmworkers in both experimental groups had significant positive changes in their knowledge. These changes were more pronounced for farmworkers in experimental group #1 (for experimental group #1: sum of squares [SS] = 3142.89, F = 135.60, p < .001; for experimental group #2: SS = 514.57, F = 22.35, p < .001). Moreover, for farmworkers in experimental group #1, the positive changes in

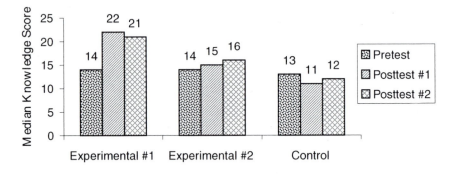

FIGURE 4.2. Median Knowledge Index Scores

knowledge persisted over time (i.e., at posttest #2) (for experimental group #1: SS = 120.01, F = 5.6, p < .05; for experimental group #2: SS = 59.11, F = 3.4).

Sexual Activity

Figures 4.3 and 4.4 present data on sexual activity at the three assessments. During the month prior the pretest survey, slightly more than one-third of the farmworkers in each of the study groups were sexually active (Figure 4.3). The proportion of sexually active farmworkers showed little change between the pretest and posttest #1 surveys (one-month period) and between the posttest #1 and posttest #2 surveys (three-month period). Moreover, at each of the three time points, the majority of the sexually active farmworkers had had sex with a sex worker (Figure 4.4).

Condom Use During Sex with a Sex Worker

During the one-month period between the pretest and posttest #1 surveys, we observed dramatic changes in the reported condom use behavior of farmworkers in experimental groups #1 and #2 (Figure 4.5). For instance, compared with three out of twenty-six sexually ac-

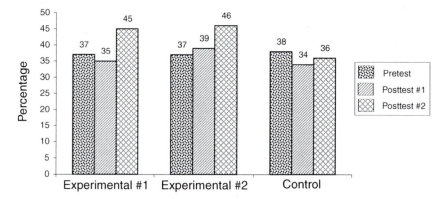

Note: The sample sizes of sexually active farmworkers were as follows: experimental group #1 (N = 85): pretest = 31, posttest #1 = 30, posttest #2 = 38; experimental group #2 (N = 96): pretest = 35, posttest #1 = 37, posttest #2 = 44; control group (N = 90): pretest = 34, posttest #1 = 31, posttest #2 = 32.

FIGURE 4.3. Sexually Active Farmworkers

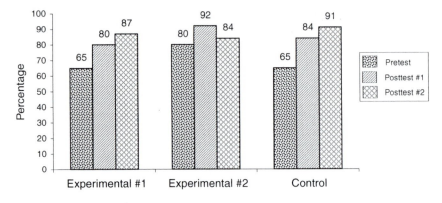

Note: The sample sizes of sexually active farmworkers who had sex with a sex worker were as follows: experimental group #1: pretest = 20/31, posttest #1 = 24/30, posttest #2 = 33/38; experimental group #2: pretest = 28/35, posttest #1 = 34/37, posttest #2 = 37/44; control group: pretest = 22/34, posttest #1 = 26/31, posttest #2 = 29/32.

FIGURE 4.4. Sexually Active Farmworkers Who Had Sex with a Sex Worker

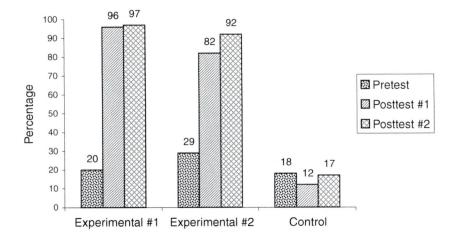

Note: The posttest #2 sample sizes of sexually active farmworkers who had sex with a sex worker and used a condom were as follows: experimental group #1 = 32/33; experimental group #2 = 34/37; control group = 5/29.

FIGURE 4.5. Condom Use During Sex with a Sex Worker

tive farmworkers in the control group, twenty-three out of twenty-four sexually active farmworkers in experimental group #1 and twenty-eight out of thirty-four sexually active farmworkers in experimental group #2 used a condom during sex with a sex worker. Furthermore, the positive change in safer-sex practices remained relatively stable over time as reflected in the proportion of farmworkers in the two experimental groups who had sex with a sex worker and used a condom at posttest #2 (about three months after posttest #1).

During the month prior to the pretest survey, very few farmworkers in the three study groups used a condom during sex with a sex worker. For instance, only four out of twenty sexually active farmworkers in experimental group #1 and eight out of twenty-eight sexually active farmworkers in experimental group #2 compared with four out of twenty-two sexually active farmworkers in the control group used a condom.

Facilitators of Behavior Change

Several factors were credited with helping farmworkers change their behavior. These factors included the information presented in the educational programs, concerns about their health, social norms as practiced by their friends, family responsibilities, the cost of health care, and, issues specific to the use of condoms.

According to the farmworkers, the educational programs provided them with information on the consequences of HIV infection and ways to protect themselves. This information offered them reasons to change their behavior:

- The *fotonovela* and the *radionovela* [for farmworkers] showed what could happen [if we did not use a condom] and that is why we decided to use condoms.
- I had little information [prior to the educational program] and now that I know a little more, I always try to use them [condoms] with prostitutes and other people that I do not know very well.
- The program motivated us to take protection since we saw the risks we were taking.
- I knew about condoms in Mexico but used them only when the prostitutes asked to do so. The program here has motivated me to use them regularly.

- Based on what I saw in the program, I now use condoms even if the prostitute does not insist that I use them.
- By listening to the *radionovela* for farmworkers I learned that it is better for yourself [to use a condom] so as not to get sick, since when you do not know you do not do it for that reason.
- The fact that the program explained a little more about condoms to us, and that made me reconsider and think more about protecting myself.

Farmworkers said they could relate to the characters portrayed in the educational materials, which further reinforced their motivation to follow the healthy course of action prescribed in the materials. As some farmworkers stated,

- Seeing that Sergio got sick and that his life was about to end. When one sees that that happens [due to HIV] you would not want to be in his place.
- Seeing how Sergio was told that his family was sick of AIDS, knowing that, motivated me to protect myself.

Concerns for their and their families' health were other reasons for farmworkers to change their behavior and reduce their risk profile. The decision to act on these concerns and use a condom during sex with a sex worker is reflected in the following statements by some of the farmworkers,

- The main thing is to stay alive; that is why I use a condom.
- By using a condom I avoid being sick.
- The expense of cures could cost more than one-hundred dollars if I get infected.
- We now use condoms because of the health concerns of our families that are left in Mexico.
- Even though I am single, I now use a condom just like my friends who are married because some day I plan to have a family.

Peer pressure was another reason why many farmworkers started using a condom during sex with a sex worker. Many farmworkers started using a condom during sexual activity with a sex worker because their friends also started using condoms or because their friends started advising them to use condoms:

- I have friends who tell me to use them [condoms] and in that way I protect myself and continue protecting myself.
- My older friends recommend it for protection against sexually transmitted diseases.
- My friends told me to use them all the time since they knew about sexually transmitted diseases and I also do the same with my friends now because AIDS has spread so much.
- I had a friend who had gonorrhea transmitted to him by a prostitute and then I thought about protecting myself.

Although condom use impaired the sexual experience for some men, they said that the benefits of practicing safe sex outweighed this drawback. As some farmworkers reflected:

- It was not a problem that it took longer to come when using a condom, even though it [sex] did not feel the same.
- Although it [sex] does not feel the same when you use a condom, one gets protection.
- There is no problem getting an erection due to the use of a condom.
- Using a condom is the same as loving yourself and I do not feel less of a man by doing it.

Impediments to Behavior Change

Some of factors identified as impediments to behavior change included the lack of physical pleasure when using a condom, social norms, issues of self-image, lack of information, fatalistic beliefs, and misconceptions about disease etiology. The most important reason for farmworkers not changing their behavior was their perception and/or past experience of a lack of or reduction of physical pleasure during sexual activity when using a condom. Some of the statements stressing this point included:

- It does not feel the same. You do not enjoy it [sex] the same using a condom than without a condom; personally that is how it is. By not using a condom with a woman I feel more excitement.

- One time when I went to a prostitute and tried to use a condom, the coldness of the condom made me lose my erection.
- If a prostitute asks me to use a condom, well, I would tell them in that case it is not worth it for me to touch her since it does not feel the same.
- The truth is I went with the prostitute and yes, I did know that there are diseases out there but I did not have anything with me. Besides I had heard that it does not feel the same and I said, I am going to go like that and thought if I get the disease, well, that will be my luck.
- For me, the truth is that you get into position better without a condom.
- I would pay a prostitute more to do it without a condom; you feel better without a condom.

Another reason given was the prevailing social norms among the social network. Farmworkers who wanted to use a condom were ridiculed by their friends and made to feel like less of a man. As some farmworkers commented:

- Some of my friends would tell me to use it and others would tell me not to, what for. That way it feels nicer and so I do not use it. No way am I going to use it! Friends, like, make you out to be different if you use it; they say you are a coward [if you use a condom].
- In reality, a lot of friends say to me go with so and so and do not use a condom; it feels great and it feels like it fits better.

Self-image and the perception of manliness also played an important role in some farmworkers deciding not to use a condom during sex with a sex worker. As some farmworkers stated:

- Well, I feel less of a man if I use a condom, and I'd rather be the same as my friends who do not use a condom.
- What I want is for the prostitutes to make it worth the ten dollars since it costs me two hours of work to earn them and it feels more manly without a condom.

A certain amount of fatalistic belief existed among farmworkers who did not use a condom during sex with a sex worker. For example, some farmworkers said:

- I do not use condoms. Well, I believe that everyone dies in a manner of their own choice and you do it the way you feel best.
- There are a lot of fellow countrymen over here, so they already know the way to live here and some say go over there where the women show up and if one says with or without a condom say why since after all we are going to die anyway.
- I do not use a condom because it is God's will if something happens to me.
- I always think of the worse [when I have sex with a prostitute and do not use a condom] but I risk it. You think maybe the prostitute has it or maybe she does not and you risk it and not use it.

Some farmworkers indicated that sex workers never asked them to use a condom and that even if asked they would not use a condom. Moreover, some farmworkers were under the impression that the sex workers were healthy. For example, some farmworkers stated:

- If I went to a prostitute and she asked me to use a condom I'd rather go with another one and not use it.
- The truth is that the prostitutes check themselves in the clinics and that is why I do not use condoms.
- I would look for a woman who is not sick.
- Sometimes you know women that are cautious and they do take care of themselves. For that reason you trust you do not have to use it.
- I do not use a condom with a prostitute because if I wear a condom she is going to think that I could be sick.

Misconceptions regarding disease etiology and prevention also precluded some farmworkers from using a condom. As a few farmworkers stated:

- Yes, a prostitute asked me to use a condom but I did not use it. I think it is luck and the blood type whether you get sick or not.
- There was a certain type of weak blood in people who get sick.

Impact of the Educational Programs

Our research concluded that both programs effectively enhanced HIV-related knowledge among the farmworkers. The impact of Program #1 was much more pronounced and longer lasting. This may be due to the unique structure of the program, which incorporated the social realities of the farmworkers into the education protocol. Although gains in knowledge are important, if they do not translate into positive behavioral changes the spread of the HIV epidemic will not be slowed.

We observed a dramatic impact on the behavior of primary consideration: the use of condoms during sex with a sex worker. Farmworkers in both experimental groups reported remarkable changes in their behaviors. More important, as reflected in the reasons for changing behaviors, the farmworkers related to the programs for a variety of reasons including the information presented, social norms, family responsibilities, and issues specific to the use of condoms. All of these topics were covered in the educational programs. Reasons given for not changing behaviors may be more an indication of the limitations of the educational programs. The programs did not focus on issues of self-image or fatalistic beliefs. Future versions of the program would need to address some of the issues raised for not wanting to change behaviors.

CONCLUSION: LESSONS LEARNED

Many factors contributed to the success of this collaboration. From the academic partners' perspective, the success was due to: the high degree of visibility and credibility of the community partner (institution and staff) among the target population; the professionalism of the staff in terms of their expertise, experience, and dedication to the target population; willingness of the outreach workers to work at anytime of the day or night; appropriate infrastructure and resources to conduct multiple service-oriented programs and scientific research; realization of the importance of rigorous scientific evaluation methods and measures; the willingness to incorporate scientific methods in program implementation; respect for each partner's expertise and experience and areas of responsibilities.

From the community partners' perspective, the success was due to the academic partners' direct involvement with the outreach workers; extensive experience working with farmworkers which facilitated the working relationship with the ASO and outreach workers; willingness to educate and train the staff for every project-related activity; positive encouragement and involvement of the outreach workers during the development, implementation, and evaluation phases of the research; regularly scheduled meetings of the whole project team to define action plans, assess progress, and solve unexpected problems; and the patience and understanding extended by the academic partner.

Collaborative community-level efforts between community-based and academic institutions pose tremendous challenges to both institutions. Much effort is needed to ensure that a delicate balance is maintained between the scientific integrity (a priority of the academic partner) and community sensitivity (a priority of the community partner) of the equation in collaborative research.

Academic partners, in their zeal to accomplish their research programs, may appear to exploit their community partners, and as a result, the target population. This is especially true when the partnership is based on an unequal power structure, with the academic partner having the upper hand. The perception of exploitation may take several forms. The community partner may feel that the academic partner is using its structures and networks only as conduits to accomplish the research goals, withholding funds and not involving the community. Academic partners may harbor negative perceptions about their community partners. These negative perceptions may be due to a lack of confidence in the community partner's capability and expertise to implement, document, and gather research data which conforms to scientific norms and rigor.

If both the community and academic partners transcend the initial stages of suspicion, doubt, and lack of respect, a true collaborative partnership based on mutual respect for each partner's expertise and experience can evolve benefiting not only the two collaborative partners but, most importantly, the target population they wish to serve.

Despite best efforts, community-level collaborations are not immune to extraneous disruptive factors. These disruptive factors impacted the study implementation and affected sample accrual, cooperation rates, and attrition rates. For instance, some participants in our sample were not willing to cooperate with us because the farm owners had threatened to fire them. In another incident described earlier, one of the farm owners thought we would report him to the authorities because he hired farmworkers without proper authorization to work in the United States. The farm owner refused to allow the research staff to conduct follow-up work on his farm. When the research staff tried to educate the farm owner about the importance of the work, the farm owner's helper pulled out a gun and threatened the research staff. Despite our proactive efforts to include farm owners into our network of decision makers and community leaders, many still harbored suspicions. The concerns of farm owners about our work were primarily due to their fear that we would: empower the workers, unionize them, and report to the relevant authorities their hazardous working and living environments.

Another challenge to the study implementation efforts came from the INS. Since some farmworkers do not have proper authorization to work in the United States, the INS conducts "spot" raids in the fields and deports unauthorized farmworkers. Naturally, many farmworkers were fearful of talking to us. This fear of the INS, unfortunately, was carried over to other authorities such as medical professionals. Farmworkers are hesitant to visit health care providers even when they need care.

Through extensive efforts and cooperation we were able to address some of challenges posed in the field by intransigent farm owners and other authorities. To gain access to the sample living in campsites, we included farm owners in our advisory groups and informed them about the progress of the work. In addition, we recruited the "boss" of each campsite into the study. The boss gathered farmworkers for the implementation work, and informed us about the movement of the study sample between campsites or out of the study area. In addition, out of concerns for the safety of the research staff and the study participants, we included the INS and police in out network of authorities who we kept informed about the study.

Having transcended the normal problems encountered by most community-level collaborations, the collaborations between Vista Community Clinic and UC Irvine have been able to focus their energies toward the evolution of new strategies in terms of methodologies and technologies that address the needs of the target population. We were able to successfully implement scientifically complex and rigorous research in this hard-to-reach population. Moreover, in view of participants' low levels of formal educational backgrounds, we developed innovative, reliable, and valid data collection techniques, which take into consideration the fact that many of the study participants may be more comfortable in reading icons rather than the written word. In terms of the educational program, the materials were in a format more conducive to the target population. The materials used farmworkers as role models and actors. Furthermore, the story line developed in the materials is similar to the actual life experiences of farmworkers. Last, to ensure appropriate follow-up accrual of the target population, we developed methodologies that helped us reduce attrition loss due to the inability to recontact the study participants.

The success of our community-level collaborative efforts has provided many benefits to the community and academic partners, and the target population. The collaborative efforts have enhanced the sensitivity of the researchers to the conduct of research in the field, provided them with insights on successful strategies for program development and implementation, and access to marginalized, hard-to-reach target populations. For the community partners, the collaborative efforts have enhanced and institutionalized their research capabilities, and provided different versions of an HIV education program that is incorporated in their regular outreach efforts. The educational programs evaluated through our research have become an integral part of the ASO's outreach repertoire. The most important beneficiaries of the collaborative research are the farmworkers. Their willingness to share the most private aspects of their lives have helped us design and implement not only culturally sensitive and linguistically appropriate HIV prevention programs but also social service programs that address the more pressing issues that affect them: housing, food, clean water, and medical assistance.

APPENDIX: RECRUITMENT CRITERIA
AND SAMPLE SIZE OF FARMWORKERS

We recruited male farmworkers who were primarily Spanish speaking, age eighteen to thirty-five years, and single, or if married, living separate from their families. The selection criteria helped match the study sample with the models portrayed in the education program. We interviewed 432 farmworkers at the pretest, and 326 and 281 farmworkers, respectively, at posttest #1 and posttest #2 (see Figure 4.1). Out of the 432 farmworkers, we have complete data on 271. These 271 farmworkers (eighty-five and ninety-six farmworkers, respectively, in experimental groups #1 and #2, and ninety farmworkers in the control group) form the study group. For the focus groups, we randomly selected forty farmworkers from the two experimental groups (see Figure 4.1), based on them either changing or not changing their behavior between the pretest and the posttest assessments. Farmworkers were grouped as having changed their behavior if, at the pretest, they reportedly did not use a condom during sex with a sex worker but did so at either of the posttests.

NOTE

1. A novela is a serial story that may appear in several formats, including video, radio, and print. It offers an effective health education tool through: (1) the use of pictures to tell a story, (2) a story line that incorporates health behaviors and lifestyles, and (3) a culturally sensitive medium. The picture and audio formats, which require little or no reading, are potentially effective ways to teach low-literacy Spanish-speaking farmworkers about HIV. We had conducted preliminary evaluation studies on the efficacy, linguistic appropriateness, and cultural sensitivity of these materials among farmworkers (Mishra, S.I., Conner, R.F., 1996).

Typically, novelas use a three-model approach to convey issues involved in the decision to adopt a particular health behavior. Of the three models, one consistently demonstrates unhealthy behavior, another consistently demonstrates healthy behavior, and the primary model vacillates between the "good" and "bad" behavior. The drama shows negative consequences arising out of unhealthy behavior and positive consequences stemming from healthy lifestyle choices. As the story progresses, the primary model eventually makes a transition incorporating healthier behaviors and, as a result, has an improved outcome. The target audience, which generally identifies with the primary model, sees how this character makes a healthy transition in lifestyle relating to the health issue and is encouraged to make changes.

The *Tres Hombres* materials included both an eight-page *fotonovela* and a fifteen-segment *radionovela* (five minutes per segment). The materials told the same basic story of three men, Victor, Sergio, and Marco. Victor was portrayed as the character who demonstrated consistently healthy behavior. He was married and never had sexual relations outside of marriage. Sergio was the character who demonstrated consistently unhealthy behaviors. He was married but had a history of sexual relations with other women, sex workers, and other men. In addition, Sergio had used injectable drugs. Marco was portrayed as the primary model. He was single and was open to behavioral experimentation.

As the story continues, the three men leave their families to cross the Mexico-U.S. border to work in the agriculture fields. After work, they meet Karla, a sex worker, who informs them of the risk of HIV and how to prevent it by using condoms. Sergio refuses to heed Karla's suggestion and, in turn, Karla refuses to have sex with him. Marco, on the other hand, listens to Karla's advice. As the story progresses, Sergio discovers that his wife and new baby, who had remained in Mexico, were sick and infected with the virus. Marco, who learned to use a condom, and Victor, who abstained from sex, remained healthy. Medical personnel from both folk and modern medical traditions played roles as disseminators of the information.

The *Marco Aprende fotonovela* contained pictures that explained where to obtain a condom and how to use and dispose of it. It addressed issues of self-efficacy and imparted practical knowledge and the means to develop behavioral skills. In addition, it included a couple of condoms for practice and use.

REFERENCES

Bronfman, M. and Moreno, S.L. (1996). Perspectives on HIV/AIDS prevention among immigrants on the U.S.-Mexico border. In S.I. Mishra, R.F. Conner, and J.R. Magaña (Eds.), *AIDS Crossing Borders: The Spread of HIV Among Migrant Latinos* (pp. 49-76). Boulder, CO: Westview Press.

Conner, R., Mishra, S.I., and Magaña, J.R. (1996). HIV prevention policies and programs: Perspectives from researchers, migrant workers and policymakers. In S.I. Mishra, R.F. Conner, and J.R. Magaña (Eds.), *AIDS Crossing Borders: The Spread of HIV Among Migrant Latinos* (pp. 185-214). Boulder, CO: Westview Press.

Conner, R., Mishra, S.I., and Magaña, J.R. (1998). A model for moving science into policy: The case of AIDS prevention research on migrant Latinos. In J.H. Stanfield and E. Margolis (Eds.), *AIDS Research/AIDS Policy: Competing Paradigms of Science and Public Policy* (pp. 159-186). Greenwich, CT: Jai Press, Inc.

Marin, B., Otero-Sabogal, R., and Perez-Stable, E.J. (1987). Development of a short acculturation scale for Hispanics. *Hispanic Journal of Behavioral Science 9*(2), 183-205.

Mishra, S. and Conner, R.F. (1996). Evaluation of an HIV prevention program among Latino farmworkers. In S.I. Mishra, R.F. Conner, and J.R. Magaña (Eds.), *AIDS Crossing Borders: The Spread of HIV Among Migrant Latinos* (pp. 157-181). Boulder, CO: Westview Press.

Mishra, S., Conner, R.F., and Magaña, J.R. (1996). Migrant workers in the United States: A profile from the fields. In S.I. Mishra, R.F. Conner, and J.R. Magaña. (Eds.), *AIDS Crossing Borders: The Spread of HIV Among Migrant Latinos* (pp. 3-24). Boulder, CO: Westview Press.

Chapter 5

A Health Promotion Intervention for Prison Inmates with HIV

Barry Zack
Olga Grinstead
Bonnie Faigeles

"Are you saying that I can be living with HIV longer than my sentence . . . and not die from AIDS inside the prison?" This is a common question asked by inmates with HIV after learning more about the spectrum of HIV disease; after learning about healthy living with HIV; after learning that they can make life changes. The biggest fear HIV-positive inmates have is that they will die while incarcerated. Both of these growing epidemics, HIV and incarceration, have taken an enormous toll on our communities.

INTRODUCTION

In 1986, staff members of a local AIDS Service Organization (ASO), called the Marin AIDS Project (MAP), joined with a physician to teach an introductory course in HIV, STD, and hepatitis prevention to a class of prisoners preparing to be released. After two classes, the physician gave the ongoing responsibility of teaching the class to MAP. The staff slowly developed trust with both the inmates and prison teachers in an effort to expand educational opportunities throughout the prison. The staff was soon teaching in other educational settings, such as classes in vocational training and high school equivalency degrees. Inmates in the prerelease class urged the instructors to teach newly arriving inmates as well. The warden was very receptive. He had a classroom built for this "HIV orientation class" and required all arriving inmates to take the class. That year, over 12,000 inmates participated in the HIV orientation class.

This led to the development of "inmate peer HIV education" training. Inmates with HIV were trained to be peer educators with the goal of boosting the perception of risk among new inmates. The HIV-positive inmate educators facilitated an "AIDS Basics" class to make the point: "I didn't think I was at risk. I didn't think I could get it. I'm HIV positive today because I wasn't thinking." This project led to an increase of voluntary HIV antibody testing in the prison, which in turn led to an increase in the number of inmates identified as HIV infected. HIV-infected prisoners believed that AIDS was a death sentence atop their existing prison sentence. Clearly, an immediate need evolved to develop a program that would address the needs of inmates with HIV.

Having previously developed, implemented, and evaluated a pre-release intervention for general population inmates (Grinstead, Zack, and Faigeles, 1999) MAP developed a health promotion intervention for soon-to-be-released inmates with HIV in an effort to reduce their high-risk behaviors and increase use of community services. The goal of this project was to develop a program, assess its feasibility, and then evaluate its effectiveness. This project was conducted in collaboration with the prison, a community-based service provider, and an academic research institution. Collaboration between community-based service providers and academic researchers is becoming widely recognized as a means of reaching and providing programs for disenfranchised populations—and conducting important research as well (Altman, 1995; Bauman, Stein, and Kreys, 1991; Binson et al., 1997; Gomez and Goldstein, 1995).

After the first year of this collaborative project, the prison intervention staff at the Marin AIDS Project moved to Centerforce, a statewide agency whose sole mission is to provide support and services in collaboration with the incarcerated community. The move was designed to allow intervention staff to move beyond the mission of MAP (Marin AIDS Project). This was precipitated by two factors: (1) the desire of the inmate population to expand the educational project to include not just AIDS, but other sexually transmitted diseases, tuberculosis, and hepatitis as well, and (2) the increasing numbers of requests by institutions outside of Marin County seeking support, technical assistance, and consultation to develop similar programs in their institutions.

The transition from the Marin AIDS Project to Centerforce did not impair program activities; to the contrary, it offered enormous dissemination opportunities.

JUSTIFICATION

The number of Americans who are incarcerated has doubled in the past twelve years. As of March 2000, over 2 million Americans were incarcerated in this country's prisons and jails. Sixty percent of federal prisoners and nearly one-fourth of those in state prisons and local jails are incarcerated for drug offenses. Thus, it is not surprising that among the incarcerated, the numbers of individuals living with HIV or AIDS has also increased. A recent survey showed that the prevalence of AIDS among prisoners in the United States is five times that of the general population (Hammett, 1994). In one study comparing blind seroprevalence estimates to voluntary testing results, only 47 percent of inmates accepted voluntary testing and only 34 percent of the HIV-positive individuals were identified by voluntary testing (Behrendt et al., 1994). In 1994, a blind seroprevalence survey of inmates in California found 2.4 percent of male inmates and 3.2 percent of female inmates to be infected with HIV (California Department of Corrections, 1995). In a more recent study of inmates participating in a prerelease HIV prevention program, 6.5 percent of participants reported having tested positive for HIV (Grinstead, Zack, and Faigeles, 1999).

Because most inmates are serving short sentences for parole violations and recidivism to prison is common (California Department of Corrections, 1997), at-risk individuals move frequently between prisons and their home communities. Men and women leaving prison face multiple challenges—interpersonal, financial, and vocational. They also have difficulty securing health and social services. These challenges are compounded for men living with HIV.

As a result, recognition is growing that HIV-positive persons are an appropriate and urgent target of programs to prevent new HIV infections (DeRosa and Marks, 1998; Rotheram-Borus and Miller, 1998). Without access to drug treatment, medical treatment, social services, or even the most basic food and shelter, issues such as safe sex and clean needles lose priority, even for people who know they are HIV seropositive. Consequently, when inmates return to their sexual and/or needle-sharing partners in the community, these partners face increased risk for HIV infection. Effective prevention interventions for inmates with HIV must be developed to prevent the spread of the virus to uninfected members of the community.

The period of incarceration is an opportunity to help HIV-positive inmates learn more about the virus and to plan ways to reduce the risk of transmission after release. Interventions can be initiated during incarceration and continued after release, with the help of community-based organizations. In-prison interventions could preserve lives if they connect inmates with community resources such as drug/alcohol treatment, housing, and employment. This is especially critical for infected inmates who are being treated with medication on release from prison.

The current "transitional case management services" for HIV-infected inmates are inadequate in their provision of treatment; moreover, they offer little in way of prevention services (Health and Human Services Administration, 1995). The advantage of prerelease HIV prevention interventions is that inmates have the time and motivation to attend programs and are not yet facing the stresses of community and family reentry. Inmates struggling with addiction to drugs or alcohol are also more likely to be sober during this time.

METHODS

Research/Service Provider/Corrections Collaboration

This project was conducted within the context of an ongoing collaboration between an academic institution (The Center for AIDS Prevention Studies, University of California, San Francisco), a community-based service agency (Centerforce, a statewide nonprofit agency providing services and advocacy to prisoners and their families), and a large state prison. Within the collaboration, interventions and research projects are planned by the academic and community partners; prison staff and administrators provide feedback and guidance, particularly regarding feasibility issues. HIV-infected inmates who serve as peer educators are also involved in planning intervention and evaluation activities through their participation in an advisory committee and by periodic focus groups.

The collaboration was initiated in 1990. Since then, we have conducted a series of programs and program evaluation projects (Grinstead, Zack, and Faigeles, 1999), including an evaluation of an HIV orientation program for new inmates (Grinstead, Faigeles, and Zack, 1997), a peer-led prerelease intervention (Grinstead, Zack, and Faigeles, 1999), and interventions for women visiting their incarcerated partners (Comfort et al., 2000).

Each project has led to new projects as research findings are used to inform and develop new programs within the prison. For instance, the Health Promotion program for inmates with HIV emerged after inmate peer educators and staff noticed that inmates, once released, failed to use community resources and frequently returned to prison. It was also influenced by findings of a previous study that developed and evaluated a prerelease program for general population inmates (Grinstead, Zack, and Faigeles, 1999).

Setting

This project was conducted at San Quentin State Prison in Marin County, California, a medium-security prison for men. It also serves as the Northern California reception center for the California Department of Corrections. Approximately 6,000 men are housed at the prison. Most men stay at San Quentin for less than two years. Recidivism to the prison system is high. Over 40 percent of parolees return within one year; after two years, 66 percent have been reincarcerated (California Department of Corrections, 1997). Existing HIV-prevention programs are conducted through the prison's education and medical departments. Approximately 250 known HIV-infected men are housed at this prison. HIV testing, which is voluntary at state prisons in California, is offered to men as they enter the prison. Inmates may request HIV testing at any time. Prior to 1993, known HIV-positive men at this prison were housed together in one unit. Now they are housed with the general population or on a housing unit reserved for men with chronic illnesses.

Project Goals

The goal of this project was to develop, implement, and evaluate the feasibility and effectiveness of a prerelease intervention for HIV-infected prison inmates in reducing behaviors that transmit HIV postrelease, and to increase utilization of community services after release. The underlying assumption of the intervention is that increased use of community resources can lower HIV risk by reducing the chances of recidivism, linking participants with support, drug treatment, employment assistance, harm reduction, and other services.

The goal of the intervention was to provide information, support, and referrals for HIV-infected inmates just prior to release from prison. The intent of the intervention was to improve HIV/AIDS knowledge (including knowledge about living with HIV), reduce intentions to engage in high-risk sexual and drug-related risk behaviors, and increase intentions to use community resources. The intervention was designed to reduce sexual high-risk behavior by teaching about HIV transmission, teach and practice risk-reduction skills (condom use, needle cleaning, assertion, and communication skills), and encourage the use of existing drug treatment, needle-exchange, and social services in the community after release. Use of community resources was to be increased by informing inmates about available resources and introducing them to community service providers prior to release from prison.

Development of the Intervention

The intervention session topics and format were developed in collaboration with prison administrators as well as inmate peer educators who shared their experiences in focus groups.

The intervention topics and ideas were first reviewed by inmates who had recently learned their HIV-infected status. This was accomplished by distributing a survey to HIV-infected inmates that listed the topics mentioned during the focus groups. They were asked to prioritize the topics based on level of importance.

Because of the collaboration between the community-based group and researchers, the CBO implemented a design typically used in (academic) survey methodology. The creation of qualitative interviews, focus groups, survey development, and analysis would not have occurred without the collaboration.

Service providers from the community came to the prison to conduct intervention sessions. It had the added benefit of introducing inmates to service providers prior to release. In addition, it provided opportunities for transitional case management at each session, thereby decreasing barriers between former inmates and community resources. Each session included an oral presentation, followed by a question-

and-answer period and discussion. Most presenters also distributed written material preapproved by the prison's community resources department.

Originally, the intervention was designed as four weekly sessions over a three-week period for a total of twelve intervention sessions. In the first two intervention series, however, the three-week program was extended to five weeks as sessions were cancelled and rescheduled due to difficulties with getting providers inside the prison. These problems were due to institutional barriers as well as providers failing to comply with requests to meet dress codes and to bring valid identification. Over the five-week period of time, many participants were transferred or released and thus were not able to complete the program. During this time, the problem was compounded when the HIV-seropositive inmates were moved to a new housing location, far from the intervention site. A formal request to the warden to conduct the program in a one-week format (six hours/day) was denied, as participants would have had to miss work or school in order to attend. Though the request was denied, the warden supported a solution that satisfied all the collaborative partners: intervention sessions for the remaining series were offered on Monday through Thursday evenings for two consecutive weeks. Each intervention session was two to two-and-a-half hours in length, for a total of sixteen to twenty hours. The most important component of the alternative was a convenient new location: next door to the new housing unit.

Overall, nine intervention series were conducted. The topics of the eight sessions within each series included:

1. Project introduction/HIV information;
2. Treatment update;
3. Substance use and its effect on HIV;
4. Sexuality and HIV;
5. Inspirational speaker/pain to power;
6. Nutrition;
7. and 8. Barriers to service utilization/resource fair.

The order of sessions and specific speakers varied from session to session, depending on the availability of speakers. Sessions were occasionally cancelled and rescheduled due to institutional lockdowns or other situations in which speakers were not able to enter the prison as planned. The final two sessions of each series consisted of a "resource fair." As inmates enrolled in the intervention series, their counties of release were confirmed. The project coordinator then invited service providers from these counties to come to the resource fair. During these sessions, providers met with participants to offer transitional case management services such as providing information about the agency, making appointments for postrelease services, and providing referrals. Service providers included case management, support groups, financial assistance, legal support, and food, as well as alcohol/drug treatment programs (Alcoholics Anonymous, Narcotics Anonymous, and residential or outpatient facilities), and job placement and vocational training programs. A typical intervention series outline is shown in Box 5.1.

Even after years of working with the prison, the staff still discovers new obstacles every day. During this time California was hit hard by "El Niño." Heavy rains and/or fog routinely stopped all inmate movement. It was also at this time when California reinstituted the death penalty. Because all executions in California take place at San Quentin, both the prisoners and prison staff are greatly affected by impending executions. By developing creative interventions and solutions, the Centerforce staff succeeds in continuing to provide services despite almost daily challenges. For example, if a well-informed guard (correctional officer) is not at the gate due to reassignment, illness, or vacation, program staff must reintroduce all of these elements to the new guard for approval. If the new guard is unwilling to accept our word, she or he forwards the request to the officer on duty, so that he or she does not have to take responsibility if anything should go wrong. This is why it is important to get the support of prison administrators up front. All of these challenges were either institutional or out of our control. Other challenges came from the providers we invited into the prison. Though all providers were informed of basic rules and regulations, such as what not to wear and bring, some providers still showed up at the gate with no photo identification, the most important possession for prison clearance. This is one of the challenges of working within a large prison system. To achieve our goals we must be persistent as well as sensitive to our environment, both within the community and prison institution. These are the same basic ingredients of a successful collaboration between a research institution and a community-based agency.

BOX 5.1. Outline of Typical Intervention Series

Health Promotion Series

November 9-19, 1998 (Monday through Thursday)

Monday, November 9 Introduction/AIDS 101	Icebreaker activities and an overview of the HIV/AIDS epidemic, definitions, and methods of transmission.
Tuesday, November 10 Treatments update	Overview and discussion of drug treatment options for HIV-positive inmates.
Wednesday, November 11 Substance use and its effect on HIV	Connects the use of alcohol and drugs to HIV infection.
Thursday, November 12 Sexuality and HIV	Discussion and role-play regarding disclosure of HIV status with partners, negotiation of safer sex practices, and the spectrum of safer sexual behaviors.
Monday, November 16 Barriers to release/pain to power	Presents the personal testimony of a former inmate; overcoming barriers and reentering the community.
Tuesday, November 17 Nutrition	Presents healthy, low-cost nutritional options for people living with HIV.
Wednesday, November 18 Resource fair—Part I	Links various HIV-related services in the Bay Area to inmate needs.
Thursday, November 19 Resource fair—Part II	Links various HIV-related services in the Bay Area to inmate needs.

EVALUATION PLAN (RESEARCH DESIGN)

Health promotion program participants were recruited by (1) flyers, (2) referrals from their correctional counselors, (3) inmate HIV educators, and (4) word of mouth. Men who signed up for the program were approached and asked if they would like to participate in a research project evaluating the effectiveness of the program. All men who signed up for the program were offered participation in the evaluation study. To enroll in the study, men attending the program had to be within six months of release from prison.

Because none of the collaborative partners believed it was ethical to randomize men who had signed up for the intervention to a no-treatment or wait-list comparison group, a comparison group was formed by evaluating men who were motivated to sign up for the intervention but could not actually attend due to circumstances beyond their control (e.g., change in work schedule to evenings, imminent release or transfer). All other men who signed up for the program and agreed to participate in the evaluation were considered to be in the program (intervention) group. This comparison group controlled for motivation to participate in the intervention. Some comparison group participants attended a few intervention sessions before they were transferred, released, or rescheduled.

Participants in the intervention and in the comparison groups completed face-to-face interviews preintervention, postintervention, and were interviewed by telephone after release.

The preintervention survey was designed to take approximately thirty minutes. This survey assessed demographic variables (e.g., age, ethnicity, relationship status, number of years spent in incarceration in the past decade), preincarceration sexual behavior with committed and other partners, drug-related risk behavior, preincarceration risk-reduction behavior (condom use, needle cleaning, use of needle exchange), preincarceration use of community resources before and after HIV-seropositive diagnosis, social support and coping, and postrelease behavioral intentions. Preintervention surveys also included an eight-item knowledge scale (Grinstead, Faigeles, and Zack, 1997). The post-intervention survey repeated the knowledge scale and reassessed behavioral intentions regarding sex, drug use, and community resource utilization by asking the likelihood of these behaviors after release. This survey was designed to take approximately twenty minutes.

The postrelease telephone survey was designed to take approximately fifteen minutes. Postrelease behaviors related to sexual and drug-related risk of transmitting HIV to others and risk reduction behavior (e.g., condom use, needle cleaning, needle exchange) were assessed as well as postrelease use of specific community resources. Originally, we planned to assess participants between thirty to sixty days after their release from prison. However, only 10 percent of participants were assessed during that time. Postrelease questions address the period of time "since your release from prison." Because of the extended follow-up period, some participants had been reincarcerated. In those cases, the interviewer assessed the period of time after the incarceration in which participants received the intervention.

For the intervention group, postintervention surveys were conducted in the week following the last intervention session. For the comparison group, postintervention surveys were conducted at least one week after the preintervention survey, but prior to the participants' release or transfer from the prison. All evaluation procedures were reviewed and approved by the University of California, San Francisco Committee on Human Research.

Another outcome of this collaboration was that the program team was the same team that developed the analysis plan. All team members had input into each component of the overall intervention: the research questions, developing the intervention/program, the survey instruments, and the analysis plan.

RESULTS

Despite limitations in the evaluation design and implementation problems, the results support the effectiveness of the intervention in decreasing risk behavior and increasing use of community service utilization after release from prison. As expected, the men in the intervention group reported greater utilization of community resources and reduced sexual and drug-related risk behavior than the men in the comparison group. In contrast to the comparison group, a larger percentage of men in the intervention group had a paying or volunteer job, a smaller percentage used drugs or alcohol, injected drugs or shared needles, and a larger percentage used a condom the first time they had sex after release from prison.

Preintervention Survey Findings

Study Sample

During the study period (February 1996 through November 1998) 147 men agreed to participate in the intervention study. Three men were later determined to be ineligible because they were interested in the evaluation, not the program. Twenty-one men dropped out of the study after the preintervention survey because they did not want to be contacted for evaluation after their release from prison, and 123 men continued enrollment and agreed to participate in the community follow-up. These 123 men are considered to be the study sample; ninety-four men were evaluated in the intervention group and twenty-nine men were evaluated in the comparison group.

Demographics

The demographic characteristics of the study sample are shown in Table 5.1. Study participants' median age was 37.7 years of age. Most participants identified as African American (55 percent) or white (31 percent). Of those who had not completed high school, 20 percent had a GED. Participants had been incarcerated a median of ten times in their lives including prison, jail, or juvenile detention. Of the past ten years, the majority had been incarcerated between two and seven years. Nearly 70 percent of participants earned $15,000 or less in the year before they were incarcerated; 35 percent earned $5,000 or less.

About one-third of the sample reported working for pay immediately prior to this incarceration, and 20 percent reported doing volunteer work. Immediately prior to this incarceration, the most common living situation was in a house or apartment with a spouse or partner (30 percent). Another 14 percent of participants reported living in a shelter or halfway house, being homeless, or living in their car immediately prior to this incarceration. Fewer than half of the participants reported knowing where they would sleep the first night they were released. Among those who knew, 35 percent said they would be in an apartment or house with family members. On average, participants had known they were infected with HIV for five years and were most likely to have gotten their positive test result in prison (57 percent); twenty men (16 percent) found out they were infected during this incarceration. Only 9 percent of participants received their positive test result at an anonymous testing site.

Postrelease Survey Findings

Of the 123 participants who agreed to community follow-up, eighty-one (66 percent) were contacted and assessed after their release from prison (Table 5.2). This included sixty-one men in the in-

TABLE 5.1. Demographic Characteristics of HIV-Seropositive Inmates (N = 123)

Characteristic	Percent
Ethnicity	
African American	55
White	31
Latino	8
Mixed ethnicity	5
Asian/Pacific Islander	1
Sexual orientation	
Straight/heterosexual	66
Gay/homosexual	20
Bisexual	13
Married or in a committed relationship prior to this incarceration	63
Married or in a committed relationship now	52
Last grade completed	
Ninth grade or less	13
Grades 10-12	68
More than 12 years	19
Income in year before incarceration	
< 5,000	35
5,001-15,000	34
15,001-25,000	12
25,000-35,000	6
35,001-45,000	3
> 45,000	10
Number of past ten years incarcerated	
< 2 years	15
2-4 years	33
5-7 years	34
8-10 years	19
Number of times incarcerated	10 times

Mean age = 37.7 years
N = 123 men who completed the preintervention assessment and agreed to follow-up.

TABLE 5.2. Postrelease Community Resource Utilization by Treatment Group

	Intervention (N = 61) (%)	Comparison (N = 20) (%)
Financial aid	94	70
Housing assistance	41	65
Food or clothing	48	55
Twelve-step program	38	30
Alcohol or drug treatment	28	25
Counseling	33	15
Seen a health care provider since release	69	53
Received preventive medical care	69	50
Has health insurance	31	45
Legal assistance	10	5
Working for money	20	10
Volunteering	26	15

tervention group and twenty men in the comparison group. The average length of time from prison release to follow-up was 242 days for the intervention group (SD = 280 days) and 247 days for the comparison group (SD = 177 days). No significant differences were found between the groups in the length of time to follow-up.

Postrelease Service Utilization by Intervention Group

Community resource utilization after release is shown in Table 5.2. Intervention participants were more likely than comparison group participants to be working for money, more likely to be volunteering, more likely to have had preventive health care, more likely to have contacted legal assistance related to HIV issues, and more likely to have seen a health care provider after release. Both groups were most likely to have sought health care at a public clinic as opposed to a hospital, private doctor, or other source of health care. Comparison group participants were more likely to have medical insurance and more likely to have contacted housing assistance.

Postrelease Sexual Risk Behavior

Postrelease sexual risk and risk reduction behaviors are shown in Table 5.3. Participants in the comparison group were more likely to have had sex since release and less likely to have used a condom the first time they had sex after their release from prison. Most participants had had one sexual partner since their release from prison. More than 50 percent of both the intervention and comparison groups were most likely to have had sex the first time with as steady partner. Twenty-three percent of the intervention group and 18 percent of the comparison group first had sex with a casual partner. Three percent of the intervention group and 6 percent of the comparison group first had sex with another type of person such as a sex worker.

Postrelease Drug-Related Risk Behavior

Overall, 63 percent of participants used drugs or alcohol since their release from prison. Intervention group participants were less likely to have injected drugs or to have shared needles among those who injected drugs. The most common drugs used by the intervention and comparison groups were alcohol, marijuana, and crack cocaine. Nineteen percent of the intervention group and 31 percent of the comparison group had injected heroin since their release from prison.

TABLE 5.3. Postrelease Sexual and Drug-Related Risk/Risk Reduction by Treatment Group (N = 81)

	Intervention (N = 61) (%)	Comparison (N = 20) (%)
Any sex since release	72	80
Used condom at first sex	81	68
Used alcohol at first sex	28	18
Used drugs at first sex	35	38
Any drugs or alcohol since release	59	75
Injected drugs since release	46	67
Shared needles since release (among those who injected)	6	40
Used needle exchange (among those who injected)	19	50

DISCUSSION

This research project, which was well received by inmate participants as well as by prison authorities and correctional officers, proves that a prerelease health promotion intervention for HIV-seropositive inmates is feasible. We conducted nine intervention series inside the prison in a thirty-month period. Intervention series were multisession (over a two-week period) and involved bringing community service providers into the prison to conduct intervention sessions.

Working with numerous community service providers presented challenges. Institutional changes and barriers and other challenges within the community agency called for changes in the program design and strategy. Through successful collaboration between the community-based agency and the research institution, the intervention was able to proceed without compromising either the program or science.

The intervention was feasible because of the flexibility in implementing the program. Flexibility for addressing these needs was facilitated by the ongoing collaboration between the researchers, community-based service providers, and the prison. The funder also remained flexible. This project could not have been completed outside the context of a truly collaborative relationship between the community-based service organization and the academic research group.

Although a truly randomized design was not possible, we were able to construct a comparison group that controlled for motivation to participate in the program. This is important, because traditional evaluation models may not be appropriate for community settings where those most in need of effective programs may be reached (Altman, 1995). Collaboration between researchers, community service providers and, in this case, a prison can be useful for creative evaluation designs that are ethical, feasible, and scientifically sound. Community follow-up was also feasible.

We assessed 147 men and received permission to follow 123 of them in the community. Of those, we contacted 66 percent after release from prison. We discovered that community follow-up with this population is time consuming and requires intensive staffing; only 20 percent of participants called us and the remainder needed to be called or traced. This would be an extensive burden upon a community agency where such projects are not a priority. Typically, follow-up/tracing skills are found in research-based longitudinal studies. In addition, many men had been reincarcerated during the follow-up period. Longitudinal studies of prison inmates should be funded to provide sufficient staff for intensive tracing and follow up of participants. Those who were followed were more likely to be in a committed relationship because these men were more likely to have a stable residence. Similar findings were reported in a previous study (Grinstead, Faigeles, and Zack, 1997).

Very little is known about the characteristics of HIV-seropositive inmates. Information from this study can be used to plan programs and services for this population. For example, in this study, HIV-seropositive inmates were generally well-informed about the facts of HIV transmission and prevention as evidenced by their knowledge-scale scores. The majority of participants were in a committed relationship as they left prison. This suggests the importance of involving partners in risk-reduction interventions. An intervention for women visiting their male partners, and a component for women and men with HIV seropositive partners could be included (Comfort et al., 2000). Our findings also underline the need for transitional case management to facilitate use of community resources, especially drug and alcohol treatment. Only about 30 percent of the intervention group had contacted a drug treatment program postrelease.

The intervention needs to be replicated and further efforts to evaluate the effectiveness of the intervention should be undertaken. This program should be disseminated to other prisons and jails, accompanied by ongoing evaluation. As a collaborative research project involving a statewide agency, dissemination of this approach to other settings is more readily accomplished. The academic researchers will also disseminate results and program recommendations through academic journals and conference presentations.

REFERENCES

Altman, D. (1995). Sustaining interventions in community systems: On the relationship between researchers and communities. *Health Psychology, 14,* 526-536.
Bauman, L., Stein, E.K., and Kreys, H.T. (1991). Reinventing fidelity: The transfer of social technology among settings. *American Journal of Community Psychology, 19,* 619-639.

Behrendt, C., Kendig, N., Dambita, C., Horman, J., Lawlor, J., and Vlahov, D. (1994). Voluntary testing for human immunodeficiency virus (HIV) in a prison population with a high prevalence of HIV. *American Journal of Epidemiology, 139*, 918-926.

Binson, D., Harper, G., Grinstead, O., and Haynes-Sanstad, K. (1997). The center for AIDS prevention studies' collaboration program: An alliance of AIDS scientists and community-based organizations. In A.F.P. Nyden, M. Shibley, and D. Borrows (Eds.), *Building community: Social science in action* (pp. 177-189). Thousand Oaks, CA: Pine Forge Press.

California Department of Corrections (1995). *Corrections announces TB, HIV and Hepatitis test results. Corrections.* (Bulletin #95-012). Sacramento, CA: Public Safety, Public Service.

California Department of Corrections (1997). *One-year follow-up of felon parolees: First release to parole from prison in 1995.* Sacramento, CA: Evaluation and Compliance Division, Research Branch.

Comfort, M., Grinstead, O.A., Faigeles, B., and Zack, B. (2000). Reducing HIV risk among women visiting their incarcerated partners. *Criminal Justice and Behavior, 27*, 57-71.

DeRosa, C. and Marks, G. (1998). Preventive counseling of HIV-positive men and self-disclosure of serostatus to sex partners: New opportunities for prevention. *Health Psychology, 17*(3), 1-8.

Gómez, C. and Goldstein, E. (1995). The HIV prevention evaluation initiative: A model for collaborative evaluation. In D.M. Fetterman, S.J. Kaftarian, and A. Wandersman (Eds.), *Empowerment and evaluation: Knowledge and tools for self-assessment and accountability* (pp. 100-122). Thousand Oaks, CA: Sage Publications.

Grinstead, O., Faigeles, B., and Zack, B. (1997). The effectiveness of peer HIV education for inmates entering state prison. *Journal of Health Education, 28*(6), S31-S36.

Grinstead, O., Zack, B., and Faigeles, B. (1999). Collaborative research to prevent HIV among male prison inmates and their female partners. *Health Education and Behavior, 26*(2), 225-238.

Hammett, T. (1994). *Update: HIV/AIDS and STDs in correctional facilities.* Washington, DC: National Institute of Justice.

Health and Human Services Administration (1995). *Progress and challenges in linking incarcerated individuals with HIV/AIDS to community services.* Washington, DC: Bureau of Health Resources Development, Office of Science and Epidemiology.

Rotheram-Borus, M. and Miller, S. (1998). Secondary prevention for youths living with HIV. *AIDS Care, 10*, 17-34.

Chapter 6

The Los Angeles Transgender Health Study: Creating a Research and Community Collaboration

Cathy J. Reback
Paul Simon

Stacey is a twenty-seven-year-old transgender woman. She is originally from Cambodia and immigrated to the United States by herself in 1994. Her goal was to live an independent and prosperous life in Los Angeles. In Cambodia she graduated from college with a degree in economics. Upon first coming to Los Angeles she found a job as a bank teller. She was successfully employed for a couple of years but was fired when she decided to pursue her gender transition. In order to survive financially she began doing sex work in addition to working with a temp agency. She was arrested for sex work and spent some nights in jail. The experience scared her and it seemed she was now intent on quitting the sex work. However, she realized that the money she needs to complete her gender reassignment would come more quickly through sex work. She understands that she is always at a physical and/or health risk every time she engages in sex work. Recently, she found out she is HIV positive and she became distraught. Her depression led her to miss some work assignments from the temp agency and she was fired. Then her roommate asked her to leave. Currently, she is staying with a series of friends, moving from one to another for short periods at a time.

Janet is a forty-two-year-old Caucasian transgender woman who identifies as bisexual. Janet began to identify as a woman in childhood and, as a result, experienced emotional, physical, and sexual abuse from her father. As an adult, Janet developed severe psychological problems that led to mental illness and then heroin addiction. As a result of using unclean needles to inject heroin, Janet contracted HIV. About a year-and-a-half ago, Janet attempted to overcome her heroin addiction by entering a methadone maintenance treatment program; she is still on methadone. For the past several years she has periodically engaged in sex work. Janet has a deep-rooted feeling that no one understands her as a transgender woman and, consequently, has a pattern of moving from one social services agency to another. These feelings have also resulted in many suicide attempts as well as self-mutilation. For the past ten years, Janet has lived in various shelters, on the streets, and in inexpensive hotels.

INTRODUCTION

Los Angeles County is home to a large and heterogeneous transgender population, ranging from homeless sex workers to those who are married, living in traditional households and completely assimilated. To date there has been very little information available on the prevalence of HIV risk behaviors, HIV seroprevalence and seroincidence, or the impact of HIV prevention efforts in this population. HIV-related research studies and HIV/AIDS surveillance activities have not routinely included the "transgender" designation in their data collection forms. For example, the 1998 HIV Counseling and Testing Report Form (OMB no. 0920-0208) created by the U.S. Government Printing Office for the purpose of collecting demographic data on utilization of publicly funded counseling and testing services has no transgender designation and collects no information on HIV risk behaviors among transgenders. Despite the paucity of data, several published reports from other locales (Elifson et al., 1993; Modan et al., 1992), limited unpublished data from Los Angeles County, and anecdotal reports suggest that many in this population are at greatly increased risk for HIV infection.

In recognition of this problem, in 1996 the Los Angeles County Community HIV Prevention Planning Committee gave high priority to the collection of epidemiological and behavioral data in this population to improve HIV prevention efforts (Los Angeles County HIV Prevention Planning Committee, 1996). In addition, in an HIV prevention application for prevention and education services submitted by Los Angeles County Department of Health Services to the U.S. Centers for Disease Control and Prevention, the transgender population was identified as one of the key groups for which epidemiologic data are critically needed.

To address the need for HIV-related epidemiologic and behavioral information on the local transgender population, three community-based organizations (CBOs) that provide HIV prevention services to transgenders and the Los Angeles County HIV Epidemiology Program came together in a research/community collaboration to form the Los Angeles Transgender Health Study. Two principal investigators, one from the community and one from a research institution led the study.

STUDY OBJECTIVES

To better understand the transgender population, the study had three goals: to assess sociodemographic characteristics and HIV risk behaviors, to determine HIV seroprevelance and seroincidence, and to evaluate the impact of current HIV prevention services. By bringing together three providers of HIV prevention services for transgender individuals in the county—each of which offer services in different geographic areas and work with specific ethnic/cultural populations—it was hoped that the study group would represent the diversity of this population. However, the study was limited in that it did not collect data on people living outside the neighborhoods served by those providers, or who lived nearby but refused service.

An original objective to evaluate the three CBO's HIV prevention programs was abandoned after it was recognized that some participants received care from more than one agency, making it difficult to evaluate the quality of each agency's intervention program. Instead, the team decided not to evaluate the efficacy of the agencies' intervention programs. The overall impact of HIV prevention services for transgenders was studied instead.

During the initial development of the study, the decision was made to focus specifically on male-to-female (MtF) transgenders. The decision was based on several factors. First, although female-to-male (FtM) transgenders may also be at risk for HIV infection, it was felt that this group would be very difficult to identify and recruit given that nearly all transgender clients at the three CBOs are MtF. In addition, the principal investigators did not believe it would be feasible to do expanded outreach to recruit FtM transgenders for the study given the available funding. Second, the inclusion of both MtF and FtM transgenders would have necessitated the development of a much more complex and lengthy questionnaire because of the need to address a much wider range of anatomies, sexual identities, individual and social characteristics, and sexual risk behaviors.

THE COLLABORATION TEAM

The collaboration team consisted of three community-based organizations and the Los Angeles County HIV Epidemiology Program. The three participating CBOs— the Asian Pacific AIDS Intervention Team in downtown Los Angeles, the Bienestar Latino AIDS Project in Central Los Angeles, and the Van Ness Recovery House in Hollywood—provide outreach and HIV education and prevention services specifically targeted to transgenders, serving geographically distinct transgender populations in the county.

Asian Pacific AIDS Intervention Team (APAIT)

The Asian Pacific AIDS Intervention Team (APAIT) was established in 1987. APAIT was the first Asian-Pacific AIDS service organization funded in the county of Los Angeles and has become the largest and most comprehensive agency serving Asian Pacific Islanders (APIs) in Southern California. Often, APIs remain isolated from more traditional HIV/AIDS service networks because of denial, language, and cultural barriers.

APAIT currently provides HIV education/prevention, outreach, behavior change and reinforcement services, case management, treatment advocacy/nutrition education, and mental health services (support groups and counseling). APAIT began its work with API transgenders in 1995. The current program consists of outreach, behavior modification and reinforcement groups, social and rap groups, peer counseling, and service referrals.

The agency is designed to be culturally and linguistically appropriate for API populations. The staff and volunteers represent a broad spectrum of APIs including gay, lesbian, bisexual, transgender, and heterosexual individuals, and a majority of ethnicities living in Los Angeles including Cambodian, Chinese, Japanese, Korean, Filipino, South Asian, Thai, Vietnamese, and Pacific Islander (Samoan, Guamanian) communities.

Bienestar Latino AIDS Project

Bienestar was formed in 1989 as a nonprofit organization designed to respond to the needs of Latinos with HIV/AIDS in Los Angeles County. Bienestar operates five service centers within Los Angeles

County located in the following communities: East Los Angeles, Hollywood/ Silverlake, Long Beach, Pomona, and the San Fernando Valley.

The Bienestar prevention program for transgenders operated as a satellite of the Minority AIDS Project program until 1997 when it received funding to develop an independent program. The objective of the program is to reduce the incidence of HIV infection in transgender persons in Metro and Central Los Angeles. Nearly all clients who participate in the program are Latinos and over 80 percent are monolingual Spanish speakers. The program consists primarily of outreach contacts that take place in a variety of street locations including parks, night clubs, adult book stores, and other locations where HIV high-risk behaviors are common.

Van Ness Recovery House (VNRH)

The Van Ness Recovery House (VNRH) is a nonprofit corporation dedicated to serving the needs of gay, lesbian, bisexual, and transgender/transsexual substance abusers. The VNRH was founded in 1973 and served its first HIV-infected resident in 1984. The VNRH provides a twenty-bed residential facility, day treatment, sober living, and job training. The Prevention Division of the VNRH began in December 1994 and offers HIV prevention services to nontreatment-seeking gay, lesbian, bisexual, and transsexual/transgender substance users. The services offered through the Prevention Division include outreach, counseling interventions, education/support groups, skills-building workshops, art exploration groups, transgender support groups, HIV pre- and post-test counseling, and direct linked referrals.

The Transgender Harm Reduction Program was initiated in October 1995 and is designed to reach a variety of transgender communities in the Hollywood and West Hollywood areas including persons living on the streets or in low-rent hotels, sex workers, bar queens, as well as those more assimilated and living in stable circumstances. The program consists of an outreach component and a series of four workshops designed to promote "skills building" and behavior change to reduce HIV risk. Transgender peer advocates conduct face-to-face outreach with transgender persons on the streets in identified high-risk areas and in venues such as boutiques and "queen bars" where transgender persons are known to congregate. Participants are also referred for HIV counseling, testing, and other services as needed. Concurrent with the workshops are weekly support groups, which provide a space for transgenders to discuss deeper, more in-depth issues. Job training is available to each participant after completion of the sessions.

HIV Epidemiology Program

The HIV Epidemiology Program is part of the Los Angeles County Department of Health Services and was formed in 1986 to increase the department's ability to track the HIV/AIDS epidemic in the county. The program has approximately sixty staff persons and is responsible for AIDS surveillance activities countywide. In addition, the program conducts seroprevalence and seroincidence studies in high-risk populations, and conducts a variety of other HIV-related epidemiologic studies. Several staff persons in the program have academic appointments in the Department of Epidemiology at the UCLA School of Public Health. The staff have strong linkages with the county's HIV Planning Commission, the HIV Community Prevention Planning Committee, and community agencies to ensure that high quality and comprehensive HIV/AIDS data are available for local planning and policy-related activities.

The principal investigators and representatives of the three collaborating agencies all agreed that it was imperative to meet quarterly. It soon became evident that two languages were spoken—the jargon of the researchers and community vernacular. However, as the study progressed and issues were worked out, a common language emerged with mutual understanding and respect.

STUDY DESIGN

Persons were eligible to participate in the study if they were eighteen years of age or older, lived in Los Angeles County, and identified themselves as MtF transgender or transsexual, or identified as a woman who was born male. These eligibility criteria captured the various stages of MtF transgender transition and excluded other groups of individuals that are often confused with trangenders and sometimes participate in transgender support groups, such as cross-dressers, transvestites, and drag queens. Unlike transgenders, these individuals are not in the process of changing their gender nor do they believe that their anatomy is in conflict with their gender identity (Brown, 1996).*

Four interviewers were hired for the study, all of whom were MtF transgenders and ethnically mixed to reflect the demographic profile of the clients served by the collaborating CBOs. All interviewers were trained in interviewing techniques and certified as pre- and post-test HIV counselors. These transgender interviewers were viewed as an important ingredient in building trust and rapport with the participants as well as to increase participation in the study.

Subjects were recruited for the study by prevention staff from the three participating CBOs during their routine outreach and/or prevention activities. In most situations, the interviewers accompanied the CBO staff during their intervention efforts and participants were then recruited for interviews at that time.

THE STUDY

Participants received a baseline interview and a follow-up interview six to twelve months later. Both interviews were approximately forty-five minutes in duration and were conducted in English, Spanish, or Tagalog. Participants received $15 after each interview to compensate them for their time and to encourage completion of the follow-up interview. After each interview, all participants received an HIV counseling and testing session. The HIV test was conducted with an oral fluid-based test kit (OraSure). The specimen was sent without personally identifying information to the health department laboratory for analysis. A coded identifier linked the test result to the participant for those who chose to receive their result. The HIV testing and counseling component was discussed with all prospective participants during their informed consent.

---

*For the purpose of this study, transgenders were defined as people who believe their biological sex is in conflict with their gender identity, i.e., their anatomy is male, however their gender identity is female. In addition, all MtF transgenders were eligible for participation in the study regardless of their stage of gender change (i.e., "transition"). Those ineligible for the study were individuals who identified as cross-dressers, transvestites, and drag queens—people who wear clothing of the opposite gender but do not believe their biological sex is different from their gender identity.

Interviewers offered participants referrals to needed HIV-prevention services; although potentially compromising to the objectivity of the interviewers, the team felt an ethical obligation to provide this assistance. Interviews were conducted in a variety of venues such as cafes, on the streets, in the agency offices, or inside interviewers' cars. Over time, interview sites changed.

The transgender population presents unique challenges in attempting to conduct follow-up interviews given that many live in unstable environments and, additionally, many change their names and other identifying information as they cross gender lines. To address these challenges, a variety of methods were used to track hard-to-find participants including reminder postcards and an increased monetary compensation of $25. Some interviewers traveled from one city to another within Los Angeles County to find participants for their follow-up interview. In one instance, an interviewer drove thirty miles at 5:30 a.m. to conduct a follow-up interview. Follow-up was facilitated because participants in the study were also participating in a prevention program in one of the three CBOs, which allows for ongoing contact with the agency and the interviewers. As a result of these efforts, the team was able to achieve a follow-up rate of 90 percent.

Culturally Appropriate Questionnaire

The development of a culturally appropriate questionnaire was one of the greatest challenges of implementing the study and required six months to complete. The questionnaire needed to be designed in a way that addressed the complexities of the transgender experience. For example, to ensure that questions related to sexual risk behavior were consistent with the respondent's anatomy, separate color-coded sexual behavior modules were required for those who had undergone gender reconstruction surgery, those who had not had surgery, and those who underwent surgery during the study's follow-up period. Wording of questions was carefully crafted to be understandable and transgender sensitive. Gender-specific language needed to be consistent with gender identity. To meet these challenges, substantial input was required of the community collaborators. The process was greatly facilitated by the willingness of researchers in San Francisco to share a transgender questionnaire they had developed (Clements, personal communication).

Both the principal investigators and the community-based collaborators agreed that the questionnaire needed to go beyond specific assessment of HIV risk behavior. Because the study offered an opportunity to collect vital information on this marginalized and underserved population, the research team felt a responsibility to gather as much information as possible. Therefore, in addition to collecting detailed information on sexual and drug-using behaviors, HIV/AIDS-related knowledge, attitudes and perception of risk, and knowledge of HIV serostatus, the questionnaire also solicited information on sociodemographics, living situation, use of health care and drug treatment services, stage of gender transition, legal issues related to gender transition, history of incarceration, experiences with discrimination and violence, and pychosocial issues and social support.

FINDINGS

Baseline Characteristics of the Study Group

The racial/ethnic makeup of the 244 transgenders who were enrolled in the study was as follows: 49 percent were Latin, 21 percent Asian, 15 percent white, 7 percent African American, and 7 percent mixed race/ethnicity or other (see Table 6.1). Fifty-four percent were less than thirty years of age and only 11 percent were older than forty years. Forty-seven percent had less than twelve years of formal education and 90 percent reported an annual household income of less than $36,000, including 50 percent that reported less than $12,000. Most identified their gender as female or woman (56 percent), transgender (21 percent), or transsexual (18 percent). Seventy-seven percent identified their sexual identity as heterosexual (or "straight"), 7 percent as gay, and 6 percent as bisexual. Although 30 percent reported prior surgery to enhance their gender presentation, only seven (3 percent) had genital reconstruction surgery (vaginoplasty). The most frequently reported surgical procedures to enhance gender presentation included breast augmentation (21 percent), rhinoplasty (18 percent), facial surgery (6 percent), tracheal shave (5 percent), or hip enlargement (4 percent).

At baseline, a substantial percentage of respondents reported sexual behaviors that put them at risk of HIV in the previous six months

TABLE 6.1. Baseline Characteristics of Study Respondents

Variable	N	%
Race/ethnicity		
Latin	120	49
Asian/Pacific Islander	50	21
White	37	15
African American	18	7
Multiracial/other	19	8
Age		
18-29	132	54
30-39	86	35
40+	26	11
Education (years)		
< 12	115	47
12	53	22
> 12	76	31
Annual Income		
< 12,000	121	50
12,000-35,999	97	40
> 36,000	24	10
Gender Identity		
Female/woman	136	56
Transgender	50	21
Transsexual	44	18
Other	14	5
Sexual Identity		
Straight	187	77
Gay	18	7
Bisexual	14	6
Other	25	10
Past Surgeries for Gender Presentation		
Any past surgery	73	30
Breast augmentation	52	21

Variable	N	%
Rhinoplasty	45	18
Other facial surgery	15	6
Tracheal shave	11	5
Hip enlargement	9	4
Sexual reassignment	7	3

(see Table 6.2). Fifty-eight percent reported commercial sex work. One hundred six (43 percent) reported receptive anal intercourse with a main sex partner, defined as a partner with whom they had a close, intimate relationship; of those, 64 percent did not always use a condom. One hundred twenty-four (51 percent) reported receptive anal sex with a casual partner in the past six months; of those, 39 percent did not always use a condom. One hundred eighteen (48 percent) reported receptive anal sex in the past six months with an "exchange partner," defined as a partner with whom they traded sex for money, drugs, shelter, food, or other items; of those, 29 percent did not always use a condom. These results suggest that condom use during receptive anal sex decreases as intimacy with a partner increases.

The most frequently used substances in the previous six months among the study respondents were alcohol (77 percent), marijuana (39 percent), crystal/methamphetamine (28 percent), powder cocaine (25 percent), crack (15 percent), and amyl nitrite or "poppers" (10 percent) (see Table 6.3). Fifty-three percent reported that they had been high on alcohol and/or drugs while engaged in sexual activities in the previous six months.

The overwhelming majority of participants also reported a history of needle use (see Table 6.4). However, most of this activity was related to self-administration of hormones. Sixty-nine percent reported injecting hormones, compared to only 18 percent who reported injecting drugs for the purpose of getting high (injection drug use). Thirty-three percent reported injecting other substances such as silicone or oil in order to enhance their gender presentation.

Eighty-six percent of respondents indicated that they had previously been tested for HIV (see Table 6.5). Of the 210 persons who had not previously tested positive and provided information on self-perceived risk of infection, 22 percent indicated that there was "no

TABLE 6.2. Sexual Risk Rehaviors of Study Respondents in Previous Six Months

Variable	N	%
Receptive anal sex:		
With main partner	106	43
Did not always use condom	68/106	64
With casual partner	124	51
Did not always use condom	48/124	39
With exchange partner	118	48
Did not always use condom	34/118	29

TABLE 6.3. Alcohol and Drug Use of Study Respondents in Previous Six Months

Variable	N	%
Drug use		
Alcohol	187	77
Marijuana	95	39
Methamphetamine	69	28
Powder cocaine	60	25
Crack cocaine	36	15
Poppers/nitrite	24	10
High on alcohol or drugs while having sex	129	53

TABLE 6.4. Needle Use of Study Respondents in Previous Six Months

Variable	N	%
Ever injected hormones	168	69
Ever injected drugs	44	18
Injected other substances for gender presentation	81	33

TABLE 6.5. HIV Testing, Self-Reported HIV Status, HIV Serostatus, and Self-Perceived HIV Risk of Study Respondents

Variable	N	%
Ever tested for HIV	209	86
How likely HIV positive (n = 210)		
Very likely/likely	5	2
Somewhat likely	24	11
Somewhat unlikely	15	7
Unlikely/very unlikely	85	40
No chance	46	22
Don't know	35	17
HIV Serostatus		
Positive	54	22
Negative	189	78
Indeterminate	1	< 1

chance" of being infected with HIV and 40 percent reported that it was "very unlikely" or "unlikely" that they were infected. All respondents, regardless of self-reported HIV serostatus, received an HIV test at baseline. Fifty-four (22 percent) of the respondents tested HIV positive. Among those who reported in the baseline interview that they had no chance or were unlikely to be HIV infected, 7 percent were HIV seropositive based on the baseline test.

FUTURE ANALYSES

The preliminary results confirm that many in this transgender population are already HIV infected and many others are at very high risk of infection. With the exception of gay and bisexual men in selected high-risk groups, the observed HIV seroprevalence of 22 percent is higher than in any other group in the county for which data have been reported (Los Angeles County Department of Health Services, 1999). The high seroprevalence is consistent with the general impression among many in the prevention community that a substantial segment of the transgender population is at extremely high risk of infection.

However, the availability of an objective measure of HIV seroprevalence will serve as a powerful tool for mobilizing support and obtaining needed funding for HIV prevention and treatment services for transgenders.

Additional analyses of baseline and follow-up data are planned to better define the sociodemographic and psychosocial characteristics of those in the study, the prevalence of various sexual and drug-using risk behaviors, and the factors associated with these behaviors and with HIV seropositivity. The data will also provide important information on the use of HIV prevention services by transgenders and among those who report HIV infection, and past use of HIV-related medical and other support services. In addition, the data will allow for identification of subgroups of transgenders in greater need of prevention services, such as those who report low self-perceived risk of infection and yet engage in high-risk behavior.

The results of the six-month follow-up survey will provide an estimate of HIV seroincidence among those who were HIV seronegative at baseline. In addition, the results will indicate the degree to which those who were found infected when entering the study have since been linked to HIV medical and other support services. The follow-up data will also reveal any change in risky behaviors. Given the absence of a control group in the study, however, caution will need to be exercised in attributing any observed reduction in risk behavior to a specific prevention program or intervention.

This accumulation of data should play an important role in improving the quality of HIV prevention services for the transgender population in the county. Local community-based organizations that provide prevention services to transgenders will be able to use the data to better understand the needs of this group and to tailor interventions to meet these needs. For example, the survey results indicate that many of the study respondents identified as "woman" or "transgender and heterosexual," and yet have male genitalia. This discordance between anatomy and identity has implications for HIV transmission as many MtF transgenders have reported that their heterosexual male partners prefer preoperative transgender sex partners. In addition, a high percentage of transgenders report commercial sex work as a main source of income, highlighting the importance of investing in interventions that promote alternative employment opportunities, such as skills-building workshops, job training, and job referrals (Reback and

Lombardi, 1999). The high prevalence of risky sex behavior among main and casual partners also underscores the need for prevention interventions that address sexual risk behavior in these relationships as well.

The data will inform the general HIV service community and policymaking groups about the unique circumstances and needs of the transgender population. Increasingly, epidemiologic data are used to drive decisions as to how to best allocate resources for HIV prevention services for various at-risk subpopulations. The results of the survey will allow advocates for the transgender population to lobby more effectively for resources to support HIV prevention and treatment needs. In addition, widespread dissemination of the data will increase awareness among local service providers to the needs of the transgender population, increasing the likelihood that services will be designed to meet their needs. The data will also help identify barriers to HIV prevention, medical treatment, and social services among transgenders, and identify strategies to improve linkages between these services.

BENEFITS AND CHALLENGES OF COLLABORATION

Conducting a research-community collaboration presented many challenges. From the onset, both the researchers and the community collaborators agreed that rather than hiring interviewers from the research institute's pool, interviewers would be recruited from the community and then trained. However, during the course of the study it became apparent that transgender interviewers were more likely to become emotionally invested in the study participants. For example, in one situation an interviewer confronted agency program staff regarding the nature of that agency's transgender services. The principal investigators were called in to resolve the conflict.

Although it was agreed that the ideal way for the interviewers to gain access to the population was through the agency staff, problems arose because the interviewers were not employed and trained by the participating agencies. During one evening outreach shift in which an interviewer accompanied two transgender outreach workers, the interviewer found herself harassed by an intoxicated drug abuser and had difficulty extricating herself from the situation. The following day the interviewer and outreach workers met with one of the principal investigators and it became clear that, although trained in interviewing techniques, the interviewers were not trained in strategies of fieldwork including outreach safety procedures. As a result, study operations had to be modified to ensure greater safety.

Many benefits of the collaborative research process were realized during the course of the project. Prior to the onset of the study, the three participating community agencies had relatively little contact. However, during the planning and implementation of the study, ongoing communication was required of collaborators from each of the agencies. As a result of this frequent interaction, a rapport was established between agencies that has allowed for better coordination of services as well as sharing of information regarding programs and interventions. Since the completion of the Los Angeles Transgender Health Study the collaborating agencies have continued to work together and have joined forces with additional agencies to form the Los Angeles Transgender Youth Consortium (funded by the city of Los Angeles). In addition, community events such as the annual Trans Pride Festival and the Transgender Youth Symposium have been offshoots from this original collaboration. This rapport was facilitated by the decision to assign each transgender interviewer to one agency and to also allow them to assist other agencies when workload increased. As the interviewers developed a sense of teamwork and accomplishment, they became the focal point for bringing the agencies together. In addition, interviewers asserted that the mere existence of the study sent a powerful message to transgender individuals: their community is important and they should continue to organize and advocate for their needs.

Researchers alone could not have conducted this study. The researchers needed the community to access the population and to help develop a culturally appropriate study. Similarly, community service providers and members of the Los Angeles transgender community needed the technical assistance from the researchers to design the study and systematically collect data. Together, researchers, community HIV prevention service providers, and members of the transgender community collaborated to design and implement this study. One outcome of the Los Angeles Transgender Health Study is that it will serve as a stimulus for ongoing interagency collaboration and organized efforts within the local transgender community to advocate for HIV prevention and related services targeted to this population.

REFERENCES

Brown, M. and Rounsley, C.A. (1996). *True Selves: Understanding Trans-Sexualism.* San Francisco: Jossey-Bass Publishers.

Elifson, K.W., Boles, J., Posey, E., Sweat, M., Darrow, W., and Elsea, W. (1993). Male transvestite prostitutes and HIV risk. *American Journal of Public Health, 83,* 260-262.

Los Angeles County Department of Health Services (1999). *HIV Epidemiology Program: An Epidemiologic Profile of HIV and AIDS in Los Angeles County.*

Los Angeles County HIV Prevention Planning Committee (1996). *Los Angeles County HIV Prevention Plan for Fiscal Years 1996/1997 to 1998/1999.*

Modan, B., Goldschmidt, R., Rubinstein, E., Von Sover, A., Zinn, M., Golan, R., Chetrit, A., and Gottlieb-Stematzky, T. (1992). Prevalence of HIV antibodies in transsexual and female prostitutes. *American Journal of Public Health, 82,* 590-592.

Reback, C.J. and Lombardi, E. (1999). HIV risk behaviors of male-to-female transgenders in a community-based harm reduction program. *The International Journal of Transgenderism, 3,* 1,2.

Chapter 7

Critical Collaborations in Serving High-Risk Women: The PHREDA Project

Geraldine Oliva
Jennifer Rienks
Lisa Netherland

I went in and was having real bad pains inside, in my stomach and in my cervix, and I couldn't walk . . . and my cousin had to carry me in, put me in a wheelchair. And when they seen tracks on my arms, doctors . . . male doctors, they were saying it's her imagination. She's on drugs. And then the female doctor came in and said no this is an emergency. My temperature was 105, and they found out I had disseminated gonorrhea . . . they kept me in the hospital for a couple weeks. But they were just gonna leave.

Focus Group Participant, 1989

Women at highest risk for contracting and transmitting HIV are poor, nonwhite, and struggling with multiple social and economic problems. Because these women have difficulty accessing and utilizing health care, they are at increased risk of unintended pregnancy and sexually transmitted diseases.

Creation of the Perinatal HIV Reduction Education Demonstration Activities (PHREDA) Project in San Francisco, California—a collaborative project between the San Francisco Department of Public Health, the University of California at San Francisco, and five nonprofit community agencies—was inspired by the recognition that a broad array of strategies are needed to reach this vulnerable popula-

tion of women with information, education, counseling, and reproductive health services.

PHREDA's primary goal was to lower the incidence of new HIV
infection in women at the greatest risk for HIV transmission and unintended pregnancy: injection drug users, partners of high-risk men,
and sex industry workers. A second goal was to prevent unintended
pregnancy and perinatal HIV transmission in women already infected
with the virus.

In this chapter, we start with a brief background on PHREDA, then
describe the three phases of the project. We include a summary of the
collaborative organization and highlights of our main research findings from each phase. We also explore how differences in the collaborative organization, decision-making and research protocols contributed to the project's successes and failures. Finally, we discuss the
unique challenges and benefits of a collaborative approach to reaching women at high risk for HIV. Through the sharing of our experiences, we hope to offer insights, suggestions, and encouragement to
others attempting a collaborative approach to their community-based
research.

BACKGROUND

I was working as director of Family Health at the San Francisco
Department of Public Health. Every day I heard about new cases
of and deaths from HIV in gay men, some of who were friends. I
read about the rapid spread of HIV among heterosexual women
in New York City and Newark and the increasing number of
HIV-positive babies who needed to be placed in foster care
there. Knowing that our county family planning programs were
not reaching the highest-risk women, I became alarmed about
the potential for the same scenario in the West. I began meeting
with community-based organizations and UCSF faculty to discuss how we could confront this issue. We established
PHREDA with a consensus that we had to do whatever was necessary stop the epidemic in women before it got out of control.

Geraldine Oliva, Principal Investigator

The project began with the observation by Dr. Oliva and her staff
from the Perinatal and Family Planning programs at San Francisco's

Department of Public Health (SFDPH) that despite the wide availability of low-cost or free family planning services in the city, few high-risk women seemed to take advantage of them. A network of family planning clinics funded by a combination of federal Title X and state Title XX dollars had ongoing funding and the mandate to provide services to this group of women. However, a survey of women attending these "traditional" family planning clinics in 1987-1988 revealed that only a very small proportion had recognizable risk factors for HIV (Darney et al., 1989). A baseline seroprevalence study of women in San Francisco showed that HIV infection rates were very low in family planning clinics (0.3 percent) compared to women attending STD clinics (2 percent) abortion clinics (4 percent), women in drug treatment programs (15 percent), and sex workers (4 percent) (San Francisco Department of Public Health, 1990).

Community meetings were held and included nonprofit community agencies providing some type of women-focused services to low-income minority populations, SFDPH staff, faculty from the University of California at San Francisco, and staff from the family planning program at San Francisco General Hospital. It was at these meetings that the PHREDA collaborative was born.

There were huge challenges in bringing together multiple institutions with different perspectives on collaborative research. The outreach staff, often women in recovery from alcohol and drugs, sometimes resisted the demands of a structured research protocol, giving priority to the needs of clients. The building the program was in burned down, necessitating a move. Coordination of many agencies required tremendous time and diplomacy. Tensions arose between staff and clients from different communities, races, and classes.

Despite challenges, the collaboration created a deeper understanding of these high-risk women, improving the quality of services and research to combat the spread of HIV. Most significantly, lives may have been saved by offering high-risk women, recruited from the streets, access to badly needed medical care and HIV prevention services.

THE THREE PHASES OF PHREDA

The PHREDA project had three distinct phases of funding and research, with collaborative partners and structure varying in each phase.

Phase One

> We're pretty much all educated on AIDS and condoms, and we're not stupid. We're pretty smart for being drug users, and that's because of the outreach workers who have reached our community. But if you had that person out there constantly, constantly getting familiar with the people and getting the confidence of the girls and all that, they'd begin to trust that person. They'd eventually begin to listen to that person.
>
> Focus Group Participant, 1989

The first phase started in 1988, when the initial PHREDA partnership was awarded the first of two rounds of funding from the U.S. Centers for Disease Control (CDC). The collaborating agencies agreed that the first step was to hold focus group discussions with the target population to better understand why they had not used the existing free family planning services, and to solicit and integrate their feedback regarding the assumptions and strategies being developed by the project. Attention was then turned to investigating ways to overcome some of the barriers that prevented high-risk women from utilizing available services. To that end, PHREDA conducted a study to determine whether targeted street outreach by peer or near-peer community health outreach workers (CHOWs) was needed—and if so, whether it would be effective in identifying high-risk women and bringing them into family planning clinics for HIV prevention and reproductive health services. The study also investigated whether women contacted by these outreach workers would be more likely to follow through on referrals and participate in follow-up care at "traditional" family planning clinics (i.e., Planned Parenthood) versus new, "nontraditional" or alternative clinic sites established by PHREDA.

Collaborative Organization

In Phase I, the project had coprincipal investigators form SFDPH and UCSF, with coinvestigators from five nonprofit agencies: Planned Parenthood, Glide Memorial Church, Bayview Hunter's Point Foundation, Haight-Ashbury Detox Clinic, and Dolores Street Community Center. The PHREDA project staff included clinic site teams, a research team, and administrative personnel. Staff were employed through a variety of different organizations, often with staff from one organization supervising staff from another organization. To provide and evaluate services at community-based organizations that had not traditionally provided these services, complex administrative and fiscal relationships had to be developed. The administrative team worked hard to coordinate activities between the contractors and subcontractors and regular meetings were necessary to ensure that things ran smoothly.

The collaborative participants also held regular meetings to make decisions about all aspects of the project, ranging from the framing of the research questions to the running of the clinics. Staff members also attended regular training sessions to enhance their skills in working with high-risk women, improve their understanding of the research project, and strengthen working relationships within the collaborative.

The collaborative nature of the PHREDA project allowed staff from a variety of institutions and agencies to participate in both creating PHREDA and its day-to-day management. The organizational structure was designed to maximize the strengths and capacities of the participating agencies. We also wanted to establish a structure that would allow the clinics started in conjunction with the project to continue operating independently after the research funding ended.

Focus Groups

In a series of four focus group discussions with high-risk women, participants identified many barriers to using available reproductive health care services. These included lack of insurance or money for health care; lack of transportation and geographic accessibility; lack of cultural sensitivity by providers; homelessness; perceived poor quality of care and experiences of discrimination and stigmatization; fear of punitive actions by the legal or social services systems; health as a low personal priority; lack of self-esteem and self-efficacy; social isolation; and lack of trust in providers (Oliva, Rienks, and McDermid, 1999).

Despite these barriers, women in the focus groups were enthusiastic about the prospect of having new services in their neighborhoods.

Targeted Street Outreach and Traditional versus Nontraditional Clinic Sites

Study Sites. PHREDA project staff selected four San Francisco neighborhoods as study sites because they had a high proportion of low-income residents, high rates of drug abuse, and high rates of STD and HIV infections: the Tenderloin, Bayview Hunter's Point, the Mission District, and the Western Addition.

To investigate whether nontraditional clinics might be more effective than traditional clinics in providing services to high-risk women, traditional clinics had to be identified and alternative clinics created. The traditional clinics already established in the participating targeted neighborhoods included: Planned Parenthood near the Tenderloin, Southwest Health Center in Bayview, San Francisco General Hospital Family Planning Clinic in the Mission District, and SFDPH District Health Center #2 in the Western Addition.

Community-based agencies already providing substance abuse, mental health or social services to high-risk women in these same neighborhoods were recruited to host new, "alternative" family planning clinics established by the project. Glide Memorial Church in the Tenderloin—which already housed a drug treatment program and many social services in its church buildings—agreed to house a new women's clinic. A clinic was also created at Dolores Street Mission, known for providing a host of social services to undocumented immigrants in the Mission District. Bayview Hunter's Point Foundation, a drug treatment and mental health center in the Bayview area and Women's Needs Center in the Western Addition, later replaced by the Haight-Asbury Drug Detox Center, also agreed to house new clinics.

Study Methods

Community health outreach workers (CHOWs) recruited high-risk women and randomly assigned them for referral to either the traditional clinics or alternative clinics to receive reproductive health care and HIV/STD prevention services. CHOWs were women hired from the target neighborhoods and trained in peer-based community health education. The CHOWs made themselves known to the neighborhood residents. They went to "hang outs" where high-risk women and men congregated and made contact with women in drug treatment facilities. Because many of the women at the highest risk are extremely isolated and not accessible on the street, outreach workers encouraged the more accessible community members to refer their friends, girlfriends, and wives to the project. Over time, some high-risk women were willing to introduce the CHOWs to or show them where to find other hard-to-reach high-risk women.

CHOWs distributed condoms and information to the people they met and introduced the activities of the PHREDA project. After identifying a high-risk woman, a forty-five-item survey instrument was administered by the CHOWs to assess knowledge, attitudes, and behaviors with regard to HIV, STDs, birth control, and use of clinical services. Women were then given an envelope containing either a list of the traditional clinics or the alternative clinics and an incentive coupon that could be redeemed for food when they came in for women's health care and enrolled in the study.

Subjects. Of the 1,438 women who were identified by CHOWs and completed the survey (the outreach sample), 794 women (55.2 percent) followed through with the referral, 384 (48.3 percent) received services at an alternative clinic, and 410 women (51.7 percent) were seen at traditional family planning clinics. At the clinics these women completed an additional 166-item questionnaire addressing perceptions regarding recent health care experiences.

The four traditional family planning clinics also allowed the project to collect data from 235 of their female clients (the family planning sample) who completed a self-administered version of the same questionnaire being administered by the CHOWs to high-risk women on the streets. Women in the family planning sample came into the clinics on their own seeking reproductive health services—the outreach workers did not recruit them. Data from the family planning sample were used to determine whether or not high-risk women were coming in for services on their own, how many were doing so, and if and how they differed from the women recruited through outreach.

Challenges. The CHOWs were recruited from the communities where they would work and were selected jointly by the project director from the SFDPH and the representatives from the CBO connected with a particular nontraditional site. The CHOWs were often women who had been clients of the CBO and drug users in recovery. Although we had a policy to hire only those who had been sober for at least six months, we had a number of CHOWs who relapsed. Some CHOWs would disappear for periods of time when they were supposed to be working. They would recruit friends for the project who would give the CHOWs some of the money they received in incentives. At first, the other CHOWs would not let their supervisors know about these incidents. Project directors only found out what was going on when things got blatant.

Consequently, we began to have regular peer support meetings with a facilitator to help the CHOWs cope with the stresses of work and to support them in their recovery. We created a periodic check-in procedure in which the outreach supervisor would page the CHOWs and arrange to meet and accompany them on their rounds. We also established a schedule of training sessions to continue to build the skills of all the staff members. Finally, the data collected by CHOWs when they had fallen out of recovery were purged to maintain the integrity of research.

The alternative clinics were established in CBOs that had been providing some type of service to very high-risk women for many years. One site was selected because of a track record in reaching "street people" in the Haight-Ashbury section of the city. This clinic had a special commitment to serving lesbian women and a tradition of making decisions by consensus involving all staff. Many staff had objections to questions on the CDC questionnaire, and felt it was biased toward heterosexual women. We shared those concerns with the CDC program officers who felt that since this was a perinatal HIV prevention project and focused on prevention of heterosexually transmitted HIV, the target population should be heterosexual women. The CDC would not alter the questionnaire, so the clinic withdrew from the study six months into the project. This caused a significant delay, as we had to identify another clinic, develop administrative and budgetary agreements, and equip the facility.

Research Findings

Overall, data analyses indicate that the CHOWs were very effective in reaching high-risk women and recruiting them into the clinics for services. The women who came into the clinics after outreach encounters were, for the most part, not significantly different from the women who did not. Furthermore, women contacted through outreach were at much higher risk for HIV infection and differed in important ways from the family planning sample, suggesting that outreach is needed if family planning clinics hope to serve women at high risk for HIV.

Comparison of Study Joiners and Nonjoiners. Of the 1,438 women recruited by the CHOWs, 794 (55 percent) came into a family planning clinic and formally agreed to participate in the PHREDA project and receive reproductive health services. Data analyses were done to compare these two groups.

Only a few differences were found between those who enrolled in the project and those who did not. Women who enrolled in the study were significantly more likely to live in stable housing (50 percent) than women who did not enroll (40 percent), more likely to desire a pregnancy, and considered themselves at higher risk of becoming pregnant in the future. The women who responded to outreach efforts were not a select group of lower-risk women but in most cases shared the same risk factors and demographic profile as those who did not attend the clinic. Not only did outreach provide education and condoms to all women reached, but significantly more women followed up by coming to a clinic for care than those who did not participate.

Comparison of Alternative and Traditional Clinics. There were no statistically significant differences in the percentages of women who were seen at the alternative versus traditional clinics (48 percent versus 52 percent), or in six- and twelve-month follow-up rates at either kind of clinic (about 38 percent for both types of clinics). This was presumed to be the result of the fact that the outreach workers met the women at whichever clinic they attended so that the women could feel comfortable and welcomed at either site.

Once the first phase of the project ended, however, and both the outreach workers and the specially trained staff at the traditional clinics were gone, there was a dramatic drop in the number of high-risk women seen at these clinics. Women who had attended the traditional family planning clinics reported that staff no longer treated them with respect, and staff reported having difficulty dealing with a drug-using population that they felt disrupted their clinic flow and disturbed other patients. In contrast, many high-risk women continued to attend the alternative clinics.

Comparison of Outreach and Family Planning Samples: Demographics. Women recruited through street outreach were more likely to be African American (OR = 3.5, CI 2.3-5.1), unemployed (OR = .24, CI .20-.29), receiving some kind of government support (OR =

3.5, CI 2.7-4.6), lacking health insurance, and living in unstable housing situations (OR = 4.1, CI = 2.6-6.5) than women in the family planning sample (see Figure 7.1).

Prevalence of HIV Risk Factors. The outreach women were far more likely to have one or more risk factors for HIV, indicating that efforts to recruit such women were successful (see Figure 7.2). They were six times more likely to have injected drugs (OR = 6.0, CI 4.1-8.8), eight times more likely to have exchanged sex for money (OR = 8.4, CI 5.8-12.2), and six times more likely to have traded sex for drugs (OR = 6.4, CI 4.0-10.3). The outreach sample was also twice as likely to have a known or suspected injection drug-using sex partner (OR = 2.2, CI 1.6-2.8), six times more likely to have a partner who served time in prison since 1978 (OR = 6.3, CI 4.7-8.5), and three times more likely to have a known or suspected HIV-positive partner than family-planning-clinic women (OR = 3.1, CI 2.1-4.8). Outreach women were also more likely to report having sex with more than one man in the last month. Despite these increased risks, outreach women

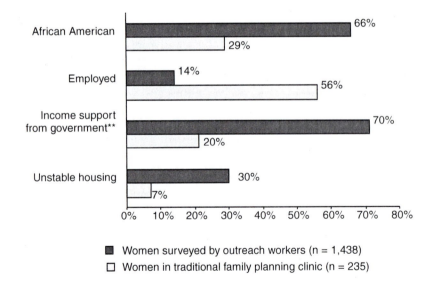

☐ Women surveyed by outreach workers (n = 1,438)
☐ Women in traditional family planning clinic (n = 235)

*All differences reported were significant at p < .05.
**Includes AFDC

FIGURE 7.1. Comparing Demographic Data for Women in Family Planning Clinics and Women Surveyed by Outreach Workers*

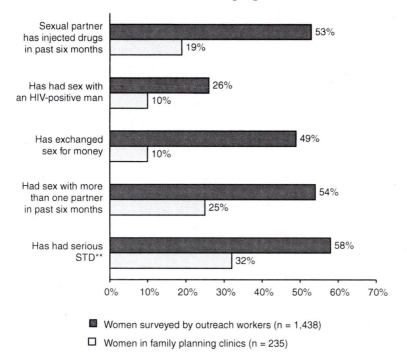

FIGURE 7.2. Comparison of HIV Risk Factors of Women in Family Planning Clinics and Women Surveyed by Outreach Workers*

did not differ significantly from family-planning-clinic women when it came to condom use, with only about 32 percent of both groups reporting doing so at last intercourse.

History of Sexually Transmitted Diseases. When compared to women found at traditional family planning clinics, outreach women were more than twice as likely to report a history of multiple sexually transmitted infections (STDs), and more likely to have had a serious STD or an STD that poses a risk to newborns (see Figure 7.2).

Drug Use History. The outreach sample reported consistently higher rates of drug usage, and was fourteen times more likely than family planning women to have used crack in the past six months. A substantial proportion of women contacted through outreach (42 percent) reported having used injection drugs since 1978, one of the primary modes of HIV transmission for women. Only 11 percent of the family planning sample reported past injection drug use.

Overall, these findings indicate that poverty, unstable housing, drug use, and sex work act as barriers that keep the highest risk women from coming into family planning clinics on their own for care. Although family planning clinics serve some self-referred high-risk women, clinic women are more likely to be employed, have stable housing, and less likely to use drugs than the highest-risk women contacted through outreach. Without targeted street outreach, family planning clinics are missing the most socioeconomically disadvantaged and behaviorally highest-risk women. In addition, more recent seroprevalence data collected by the state of California continues to demonstrate that without targeted outreach to bring high-risk women in for services, family planning clinics mainly serve women who are not at high-risk for HIV.*

Phase Two

> Da Money, da Money, da Money!! I was in a Glide drug recovery program. I had shot dope for twenty-three years. A PHREDA outreach worker came to our meeting. She was a model for us since she had been through the program. But, frankly da reason I went was da money, cause I was scared of the exam . . . lots of cancer in my family. I got to the clinic and there was this smiling, kind, pretty woman there. She didn't mind my scarred arms and dirty clothes. She didn't shrink when she touched me . . . opening up to physical contact built a trust that helped me stay in recovery. At my last visit they said they had a job for an outreach worker. I was afraid. But I was clean for a year. The pretty counselor said, "Try it. You can do it. Just be yourself." So I took the job. It was hard. I had to be on time and there was all this paperwork . . . temptation to use drugs . . . to deal in stolen objects. When I took the CHOW training in drawing blood they passed around a bag of needles. My stomach got

---

*Data are from the State of California Office of AIDS, HIV Testing Special Report, April 2, 1997, All Family Planning Contractors—Women Only Testing Services Only, July 1995-June 1996.

sick. But I had to stay focused on one thing. I needed a job to get my kids back . . . a real job with benefits. The PHREDA staff supported me and the daily check-in meetings were critical. I made it.

PHREDA client/CHOW

The second wave of CDC funding began in 1992, and funded both a clinic-based study and a community-based study. The initial design for the clinic-based study was to explore the efficacy of adding a comprehensive case management component at two clinics in comparison with routine family planning care at two other clinics. The second study sought to evaluate the effectiveness of a multipronged community mobilization effort to change community norms regarding risky behaviors and condom use in two housing projects. Our experience with the first phase had shown us that women were not following up with reproductive health care because of the overwhelming nature of their social and economic problems. During contract negotiations with CDC, the program officers informed us that this cooperative agreement would require that we change our design to be identical to other sites. This entailed dropping the case management design and instead adopting a theory-based counseling model that they felt had great potential. Theory-based activities were to be conducted in both clinic settings and in community settings.

Collaborative Organization

The collaborative organization in phase 2 was essentially the same as in phase 1. Our experiences during the first phase taught us that the CHOWs needed to be included in the regular meetings of the research team, as their perspectives and knowledge of the community could be used to improve the research. Meetings with the entire project staff were held at least monthly to review progress and to deal with problems as they arose. However, the collaborative partners did not have the same level of involvement in decision making about the research as in phase 1. Instead of framing the research question, study design, and execution ourselves in this second phase, the collaborative had to follow instructions from the CDC regarding these issues.

Using Theory-Based Clinic Counseling in the Clinic and in the Community

In the Clinics. During this second wave of CDC funding, only the alternative clinic sites were included. Because of input from the staff and community-based agencies, we moved from a traditional case-control model to an intervention-comparison model in which all clients received basic reproductive health services and routine counseling. The intervention sites would add more intensive theory-based counseling. Glide Church and Dolores Street Community Center were designated as intervention sites and Bayview Hunter's Point Foundations and the Haight Detox Clinic were comparison sites. Outreach workers recruited subjects into the clinics for family planning services including counseling and education according to the Title XX guidelines. At the intervention sites, clients were also asked to attend a series of counseling sessions based on the stages of change (SOC) model.

The SOC model developed by James Prochaska and his colleagues postulates that individuals pass through five distinct stages representing a continuum of motivational readiness for behavior change: precontemplation, contemplation, preparation, action, and maintenance (Prochaska and DiClemente, 1984). The model suggests that interventions will be more efficacious and cost-effective when matched to an individual's stage of change. Prochaska worked with the CDC to develop a manual of stage-based counseling exercises for use in the clinic.

In the Community. The community intervention (also known as the community mobilization) was based on the theory that women who are inaccessible to "outsiders" can be reached through a network of outreach workers, peer volunteers, neighbors, tenants' associations, local businesses, and family members. Outreach workers provided stage-based one-to-one outreach and prevention education, and trained housing project residents to serve as peer volunteers and deliver stage-based health educational materials. Education included stage-based role model stories and condoms, and the mobilization of local merchants to also distribute these materials. Special events for the community were also organized.

The project was designed to build a movement among residents that promoted the reproductive health of women and the well-being of their offspring. A primary goal was to have HIV-prevention messages, risk reduction behaviors, and social norms supportive of prevention behaviors diffused throughout the community to ultimately become prevalent characteristics of that community. Through the use of community peer volunteers to further the goals of the project, the community becomes both the "target" and the "agent" of change. As members of the target community, peer volunteers help shape the knowledge and norms of the community. This strategy maximizes the potential impact of the prevention education intervention.

Research Challenges

During phase 2 we again encountered clinic site problems. One of the nontraditional clinics housed in a very old building burned down after we had been recruiting clients for more than six months. It took another four months to find a suitable site in the same neighborhood. Many clients were lost to follow-up during the transition. In addition, the protocol called for specifically timed follow-up visits, so even those clients we managed to stay in touch with missed some of their visits.

Implementation of the research protocol in the clinic was also problematic from the start. Outreach workers, family planning specialists, and the clinic social workers were used to responding to the needs of each client in a personal way that gave priority to those issues the client felt were most important. These staff members were resistant to a protocol that limited the type of assistance they could provide.

Numbers, Numbers, Numbers

What I remember about the project (PHREDA 2) was the pressure to produce numbers . . . no numbers, no job. The questionnaire was too long and the clients would get bored and leave so I had the temptation to shorten the questions to the main point so I could enroll more. We got conflicting messages. Take time to carefully fill out the questionnaire . . . get more clients. But clients really liked the clinic . . . said they felt good about love, support, respect . . . so it was worth it.

CHOW

The stage-based exercises in the clinics were to be done by CHOWs, who in this project were women with no more than a high school education. Implementing the protocol required that they master Prochaska's stages, the process of change, and the stage-based exercises. This required extensive training. However, even with this training there was repeated confusion. The protocol also demanded that clients come in at very specific intervals, and this was very difficult. Our clients had been recruited from the street or from drug programs. Their lives were unstable. Many were lost to follow-up due to being in jail, the hospital, or having moved away from the neighborhood. They would often show up at the "wrong time" and we had to decide whether to serve them if it wasn't on "schedule."

CHOWs wanted to spend time with clients in the clinics and get them connected to social service agencies, medical referral agencies, or drug treatment programs instead of following a rigid protocol. CHOWs reported that clients were not interested in the exercises and instead wanted help with "real-life" problems. Other clients who had substance abuse problems would come in high and could not sit down and concentrate on a structured activity.

We had reasonably good follow-up rates at the clinics, but virtually no participants in the counseling activities. The CBO partners were angry with the CDC for imposing a protocol they did not agree with. After three years, the CDC suspended the project because they realized that the intervention was not appropriate for a population of women not in drug treatment.

In contrast to protocol implementation in the clinics, the implementation of the community intervention proceeded smoothly. However, problems were encountered in collecting the cross-sectional survey data needed to evaluate the effectiveness of these efforts. As in the first phase of the project, we had hired outreach workers from the target communities, most whom were drug users in recovery with little work experience and no research experience. A number of them had relapses during the project, and it took a while for this to be discovered.

After conducting site visits, accompanying outreach workers into the field, and reviewing completed surveys, the CDC determined that some of the outreach workers were not adequately administering the survey. In addition, a review of the surveys showed that in some instances, the CHOWs had fabricated survey responses. This situation resulted in the CDC ending funding for this study. In analyzing the problems, it was found that the supervisory staff was overextended due to limited funds and had not been able to adequately supervise the workers.

Research Findings

For the clinic-based project, we were able to recruit 301 women into the intervention and 243 women into the comparison sites. Follow-up rates for the family planning visits at six months were 64 percent for the intervention sites and 51 percent for the comparison sites. However, virtually no clients completed the minimum required visits for the theory-based counseling so we were not able to evaluate its impact and concluded that this type of intervention was not appropriate for drug-using women or for women without stable housing situations.

In the community mobilization project, the intervention was well received and appreciated by the participants in the housing projects. Outreach workers made over 3,000 contacts to provide educational materials and condoms. Many women were trained as peer volunteers and reported distributing condoms at all hours of the day and night. Local merchants distributed numerous role model stories and also provided free condoms. Special events and house parties were also held and well attended.

Problems were discovered with some of the quantitative data collected, so it was decided that a qualitative study with a sample of thirty peer volunteers should be conducted (Downing et al., 1999). These volunteers indicated that they had joined the project for a variety of reasons, including an opportunity to contribute to the community, boredom, lack of knowledge about HIV/STDs, and personal experience with STD infection or with family or friends who had HIV/AIDS. Through participation in the project, these women gained extensive knowledge about HIV/STDs and safer-sex practices. Peer education activities boosted volunteers' own self-esteem. As one participant stated:

> PHREDA helped a lot because not only do they tell you to go and pass condoms out, you know, they teach you how to present yourself, how not to be afraid, how to approach the individual. . . . And PHREDA told me how to go out and present myself to help another individual to keep from dying and they gave me that and I

used what they taught me. They didn't tell me to be mean, they didn't tell me to be so aggressive, or even aggressive, but protect myself and help them protect themselves and that what PHREDA gave me.

Interviewees also reported that the condoms they distributed were a major benefit of the intervention to the community. Several peer volunteers emphasized that most community members would not use their own money to purchase condoms. Many volunteers reported community members coming to their homes at all hours of the day and night in search of the free condoms, advice, or information.

Phase Three

The third wave of funding (1995-1997) came from the University-wide AIDS Research Program (UARP). In this study, UCSF partnered with Planned Parenthood Golden Gate, Glide Memorial Church, and Bayview Hunter's Point Foundation. The research questioned (1) Prochaska's stages of behavior change (SOC) for condom use and whether getting yearly checkups were related to rates of HIV and other STDs; and (2) if SOC-based follow-up schedules could improve client continuation rates.

Collaborative Organization

The organizational structure was far more compact during phase 3. The coprincipal investigators were from UCSF and Planned Parenthood Golden Gate. The research staff was employed by UCSF and the outreach and clinic staff were employed by Planned Parenthood. However, the UCSF staff was very involved in training and functional supervision of the staff who conducted the outreach and follow-up activities; they also administered surveys and collected lab information. Unlike the research grant in phase 2, which involved the implementation of a rigid CDC protocol, Planned Parenthood and UCSF worked together on the survey design, development, and implementation of the protocol.

Use of a Stages of Change-Based Assessment Tool
to Guide Intensity of Clinic Follow-Up

Although the SOC counseling sessions proved unworkable with high-risk women during phase 2, PHREDA staff wanted to know if an assessment tool based on the SOC could be utilized to help health care providers more effectively target limited outreach and intervention resources toward women who need them most. An assessment tool was developed that measured SOC for use of birth control, condoms, and reproductive health services. Questions about high-risk sexual behavior and drug use were also included in the assessment questionnaire.

One hypothesis was that women who were not regular users of birth control and condoms or who had not regularly received reproductive health services were in need of the greatest amount of outreach and follow-up. A second hypothesis was that women in earlier stages of change (i.e., less use of birth control, condoms, and reproductive health services) would also have higher rates of infection with STDs than women with higher SOC scores.

To test these hypotheses, women at high risk for HIV were recruited into two nontraditional clinics. The clinic at Glide Memorial Church served as the intervention site and the clinic at the Bayview Hunter's Point Foundation was the comparison site. Women at both sites were to have full clinical exams and surveys at enrollment, and at six and and twelve months. Women enrolled at the intervention site would receive additional contacts based on their SOC.

Challenges

Initially, we had proposed that clients at each site be randomized into experimental and control groups. The clinic staff and outreach workers for these sites felt that it was not "fair to randomize women" and that they would have a problem giving different levels of care to women based on some randomization procedure. Therefore, we selected two of the nontraditional clinics in communities that were similar in racial composition and degree of poverty.

One of the primary collaborators on this project, Planned Parenthood, underwent significant changes during the course of the study and merged its San Francisco affiliate with over twenty other clinics.

A change of administration and a number of staff reassignments took place in the clinics. This resulted in two severe consequences to the research project. One of the key relationships at the intervention site in the Tenderloin was with Glide Memorial Church, which housed the nontraditional clinic. The Planned Parenthood administration inadvertently made decisions about the clinic without consulting Glide. This alienated the administration of Glide, which then decided to close the clinic after the first year of the two-year research protocol.

This meant that we needed to identify another site in the neighborhood to continue the research project. Unfortunately, when the clinic at Glide closed, a new clinic location had not yet been identified and we were unable to immediately refer clients to a new site. Three months passed before a new clinic located at Milestone, a drug treatment facility, opened. During that time, outreach workers tried to check in with the clients and let them know that the clinic was moving, but no follow-up surveys or exams could be conducted. This had a major detrimental impact on follow-up rates. Many of the subjects enrolled at the original site were never located again. Consequently, we had to change the evaluation design from monitoring compliance with a fairly rigid schedule of follow-up visits to examining the impact of differing numbers of follow-up contacts.

The closing of the Glide clinic was hard on the morale of the clinic staff, particularly the outreach workers. The outreach workers felt that by closing the clinic without a replacement, Planned Parenthood had abandoned its commitment to serve these clients. The outreach workers contacted their union representatives, who immediately started circulating a flyer accusing Planned Parenthood of abandoning the Glide clients.

Due to uncertainty about how the merger would affect their jobs and the frequent changes in supervision for the CHOWs and the clinic staff, workers became insecure about their jobs and morale sank. CHOWs that had been functioning well began to misplace forms. Clinic assistants who felt pressured would neglect to do all of the required lab work or draw blood on all participants. University staff had to assume a supervisory role and also provide advocacy and support for the staff. After repeatedly meeting with the staff to discuss the problems, a project assistant for the university was assigned to be in the clinic to assure that the protocol was being followed and to do some of the paperwork during busy clinic hours.

Finally, in the last twelve months of the project, Planned Parenthood was able to assign a more senior staff person to the clinic who worked closely with the research staff to salvage the project.

> Communication and coordination with a competent manager/supervisor at the CBO is essential. In my experience, I came to the project as the manager about one year into the study. Unfortunately, there had been a lack of communication during the merger of four Planned Parenthoods, each with multiple clinics. Staff had gotten very confused about service delivery, surveys, and protocols. From Planned Parenthood's perspective, the services to the clients were being provided via several funding sources with slightly differing protocols for each source (UARP, California State Office of Family Planning, federal Title X, etc.). Staff had become unclear about which funding source covered the client and thus which services were to be provided. Due to this confusion, many clients were not receiving the appropriate services for the UARP project and had to be called back in or located again; a difficult feat in working with such a transient population. Clients had to return for missed HIV blood draws, syphilis screenings, three-month follow-up questionnaires or annual surveys and had to be given additional incentives, thus increasing the costs of the project. Many clients could not be located to return and therefore had missing data. It had become chaotic without the communication, organization, and direction of an effective supervisor who could foster teamwork among the staff.

> (Lisa Netherland, Planned Parenthood Golden Gate)

Research Findings

Study participants (n = 327) in the this third phase were primarily African-American women (71.5 percent), ages sixteen to fifty-six. Most (73.5 percent) reported welfare, AFDC (Aid to Families with Dependent Children), or general assistance as their main source of financial support and many (63.1 percent) had no health insurance. The majority (82.5 percent) were in the precontemplation (PC) or contemplation (C) stage of change (53.3 percent were not regularly using birth control, 81.7 percent were not consistently using condoms, and 51.6 percent were not having yearly women's health care checkups).

Data analyses indicated that SOC for condom and reproductive health service use was not significantly correlated with the presence of sexually transmitted infections and should not be used to determine the need for STD screening. One explanation for the presence of STDs in women who said they had consistently used condoms for the past six months is that women with STDs are often asymptomatic and may have been infected prior to initiating consistent condom use.

A significant difference in the overall follow-up rates between the control group and the experimental group was found (22 percent of subjects in the control group compared to 36 percent in the experimental group, p < .01, OR = 1.9, CI 1.4-3.2), indicating that the additional contacts provided to the experimental group improved follow-up. A further examination of follow-up rates by experimental group and stage of change (see Figure 7.3) reveals that women in the precontemplation/contemplation stage in the experimental group had a significantly higher follow-up rate than women in that stage in the control group (p < .04, OR = 1.79, CI 1.02-3.14). For women in the

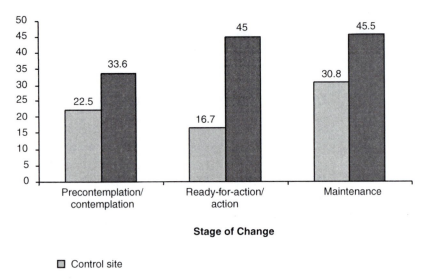

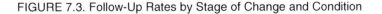

FIGURE 7.3. Follow-Up Rates by Stage of Change and Condition

ready for action/action stage of change, the differences between experimental and controls were in the expected direction and almost significant (p < .07, OR = 7.5, CI .86-64.96). No significant differences were found between experimental and control groups for women in the maintenance stage, with 31 percent in the control group returning for follow-up compared to 38 percent in the experimental group.

Logistic regression using follow-up as a dependent variable revealed that older women who lived in stable housing, had been treated for an STD in the past year, and who received multiple contacts from outreach workers were the most likely to return for follow-up (–2 Log Likelihood = 80.75, p < .0001; R2 = .25; C = .814; Hosmer-Lemeshow). In contrast, younger women living in unstable housing situations, who were not diagnosed with an STD in the past year, and who had few or no contacts with outreach workers were the least likely to return for follow-up visits. Doing an assessment of stages of change is useful in tailoring follow-up schedules, however, due to low overall follow-up rates, additional pilot testing is recommended to confirm these results.

Another interesting finding that emerged with regard to sexually transmitted infections was the positive correlation between treatment for an STD in the past year and stage of change for condom use with a main partner (r = .24, p < .001). Women who reported a higher level of condom usage in the past six months were also more likely to have had an STD in the past year.

BENEFITS AND CHALLENGES OF COLLABORATION

Benefits to the Community

From the first planning meeting, the community-based organizations (CBOs) argued for the use of nonprofessional indigenous members of the target community as outreach workers. Over time, this process created a group of trained lay health educators who would remain in the community as a resource after the research project ended.

The CBOs also argued for clinics at alternative sites, including drug treatment centers. This gave the high-risk women, such as those in drug treatment, much easier access to medical care and HIV prevention services. It also introduced drug-using women recruited through street outreach to drug treatment programs.

Benefits to the Community-Based Organizations

Planned Parenthood gained experience in serving a high-risk population and made contact with other community-based organizations (CBOs). Working with such high-risk women helped Planned Parenthood recognize the need for providing these women with a more comprehensive set of services. Planned Parenthood and the other CBOs also obtained training and experience in conducting a research study.

An important, often-overlooked benefit of the collaboration was the complementary effect produced by multiple agencies sharing resources to enhance the performance of all involved. This was done by joint trainings, sharing of space and materials, sharing of part-time staff, and coordination of services and activities to avoid duplication of effort. Agencies maximized their effectiveness in advocating for their communities at the governmental level by combining forces. Joint fund-raising and grant proposals increased the resources available to generate high quality proposals as well as increased the marketability of programs by demonstrating widespread community support for the proposed programs.

Benefits to the Department of Public Health

The DPH gained the ability to target services toward those at highest risk, thereby more effectively combating the spread of HIV. They also got exposure to the experience and wisdom of the CBOs in working with diverse communities previously not adequately served by public health or other traditional family planning agencies. Due to this experience, the DPH now colocates family planning services in its homeless and STD programs.

Benefits to the University

The university was able to have access to a population for conducting research that it had not effectively worked with in the past. The input from the CBOs and the DPH in terms of appropriate staffing and outreach techniques made it feasible to recruit and maintain high-risk women in a setting where the study could be conducted. Researchers also learned the wisdom of consulting the target community and CBOs in developing designs that could succeed.

Research staff learned that to be successful, intervention must be tailored to a targeted community rather than imposed and "forced" on the population. Researchers also recognized that there is not a magical solution to a complex problem that can be solved by one theory implemented in a rigid manner. The community had stated from the beginning that no intervention would be effective if it did not include dealing with the nitty-gritty day-to-day concerns of this population. However, the rigidity of the CDC protocol would not allow this approach. Only through the collaborative process fostered by the UARP project was PHREDA able to begin to respond appropriately to the needs of its particular target population.

CHALLENGES TO RESEARCH

In collaborative research projects like PHREDA, you've got to teach clinic and outreach staff about research, how and why it's done, and the importance of following protocols. By helping them to realize how research findings can be applied to shape policy and improve the lives of women all over the country at high risk for HIV, staff members understand the importance of accurate record keeping and following procedures. They understand what's going on behind the mountains of paperwork.

Jennifer Rienks, UCSF Project Coordinator 1996-1998

Utilizing indigenous staff, often women in recovery from alcohol and drugs, made implementation of a structured research protocol very difficult in all phases of the PHREDA project. Initially, staff did not place high value on the paperwork they were asked to generate, and sometimes misplaced or lost records. They also did not understand the critical nature of administering questionnaires in a consistent manner. They had a hard time with the skip patterns on the questionnaires and it took training, retraining, and more retraining to finally achieve consistency.

The community did not agree with the idea of experimental versus control sites. This controversy was resolved by providing some resources to the "comparison" sites. This meant that there was less money for the research component, resulting in delays in the data entry and analysis functions, which led to less productive research.

Compromise, Compromise, Compromise

> From the beginning there was tension. The CBOs wanted more and better services, the university wanted publishable research, and the county had to referee, distribute resources, and make sure that we met the CDC contract requirements. As PI, I was often caught in the middle of intense arguments. Did we need more data entry hours or more clinic counseling hours? Did we need to increase the numbers of clients seen to get the statistical power for the research sample or spend more time with clients to improve their compliance? Should we hire trained interviewers or recruit indigenous outreach workers and train them in research protocol?

> Geraldine Oliva, Principal Investigator 1989-1997

Research and evaluation are important in documenting what works and what does not work, but protocols developed by researchers often interfere with the delivery of services. The priority of staff in the clinics was to meet the needs of the clients, and the extra time and effort needed to carry out these research projects was often perceived as getting in the way.

Finally, the very nature of community-based research almost guarantees that some problems will arise. Community-based research usually takes place in the field—on streets corners, at public housing projects, or in a clinic cubicle or exam room. Unlike most true experimental research conducted in labs where the researchers have a high degree of control over all aspects of the research, field research takes place in the context of people's lives and the community. Buildings burning down and staff in recovery who relapse are just two examples of the kinds of challenges that can arise when doing research in the field.

Rather than trying to control all these threats to the research itself, the researchers and project staff must become adept at recognizing problems and be flexible in their approaches to finding solutions. This may mean redesigning a protocol that is not working, tossing out data from an outreach worker who has started using drugs on the job, or taking on tasks that another collaborative partner could not complete. Although researchers may not be able to prevent all of these problems, with a bit of experience they can become skilled in identifying and resolving problems to minimize the impact on the integrity of the research.

My Years in the Collaboration from Hell

Try juggling: (1) the clinical and personnel policies of a progressive and controversial family planning program; (2) the unique cultural environment of a powerful, inner-city, faith-based service organization; (3) the fiscal and civil service constraints of a public health department; (4) the scientific strictures and academic atmosphere of university-based research; and (5) the peculiarities and rigid requirements of a nationwide, multisite, federally funded, research intervention, and what do you get? The collaboration from hell! The PHREDA project attempted to marry the best aspects of these organizations in order to eliminate the weakest parts.

My years as the director of such a multiarm monster have left me with a set of skills that enables me to tackle almost any type of administrative, political, fiscal, personnel, program, or research challenge. But what enabled this collaboration to succeed against all odds? There is no doubt in my mind that we were successful because of the singular commitment on the part of most of the players to provide services to medically underserved and economically disenfranchised, drug-using women. Because we believed everyone was dedicated to this marginalized population, we were empowered to push through mountains of red tape and political jungles. With pitchforks, we stood in the middle of this monster that we created to hurl barriers aside that prevented us from delivering quality health care and HIV prevention to inner-city women. If I ever lost the belief that everyone wanted this to happen, I wouldn't have been able to get out of bed.

Moher Downing, MA, PHREDA Project Director,
San Francisco Department of Health 1988-1995

Administration

Collaborations among agencies with vastly different cultures present major challenges. It takes a lot of processing time for individuals to learn to respect one another's values and work styles and build the trust necessary to develop and manage a new service model. Trying to coordinate up to seven agencies requires tremendous time and diplomatic skills. Dividing resources equitably in a way that satisfies all participants again requires consummate communication skills, time, and effort. This requires a lot of meetings that take personnel from the streets and the clinics.

Dividing the financial resources makes for very complex budgeting, contracting, and accounting. This takes a tremendous amount of staff time. Again, this takes a project director away from monitoring service provision and compliance with research protocol and puts her or him in the administrative offices of large agencies. It also requires the hiring of additional staff to assist the director.

The use of peers as outreach workers and educators has been well received by the target group. However, many of these workers are themselves in recovery from drugs and alcohol and relapses among them have to be recognized and appropriately managed. Many of these women have limited job skills and education and some have not held a regular job before and may have trouble with punctuality, accountability, and the careful completion of paperwork. These staff members require sustained in-service training and close and skillful supervision.

Community

The community-based organizations (CBOs) joined the collaborative to increase and improve services for their particular target populations. They also wanted to make sure that the research conducted in their communities was ethical, fair, and of benefit to the community. The CBOs were frustrated by long and tedious research protocols that took time and resources and were not "user friendly." They were forced to learn the language of research and to demand an equal say in decisions. This meant having to develop the assertiveness and confidence to take on university and health department staff who were used to being in charge and calling the shots. In some cases, the CBOs were forced to accept research designs developed thousands of miles away by professionals who did not understand their communities.

The CBOs often carried the burden of recognizing and calling attention to tensions that arose from race and class differences among staff from different institutions and between staff and clients. Although these situations were stressful for everyone, the CBOs felt the most pressure for seeing that these issues were fairly addressed and resolved.

CONCLUSION

The PHREDA collaborative provided an important opportunity for researchers to gain a deeper understanding of women at high risk for HIV while providing much needed medical and social services to these women. The linkage between community-based organizations and traditional, Title X-funded family planning clinics has been successful in San Francisco. Many of the medically underserved, high-risk women enrolled in PHREDA continue to be served at these clinics because each of the "mother" sites have made a commitment to provide those services in their alternative clinics.

Current Status

With the conclusion of the CDC-funded research project, the alternative clinics started by PHREDA sought ongoing funding. Haight-Ashbury Detox Clinic received ongoing funding from a nonprofit foundation. Glide Memorial Church developed a partnership with Catholic Healthcare West, a nonprofit health care group, to establish a comprehensive clinical program on site. Planned Parenthood continued services at the Bayview Hunter's Point Foundation and at Milestones Clinic, a drug rehabilitation program in the Tenderloin. Both Planned Parenthood clinics are supported through grants from the California Department of Health Services Family Planning Program. The only alternative clinic that has not continued service was in the Mission District. The UCSF-administered family planning clinic at SFGH established a satellite clinic that they feel will serve the same population.

Many of the agencies that participated in the PHREDA project and had participated in the CDC-funded efforts for women in other counties are attempting to establish an ongoing collaborative network called the Bay Area Women's Health Coalition (BayWHAC). The goal of this group is to continue the collaborative interagency training, advocacy, fund-raising, and research activities that had been coordinated by the PHREDA project.

REFERENCES

Darney, P., Myhra, W., Atkinson, E.S., and Meier, J. (1989). Sero-survey of human immunodeficiency virus infection in women at a family planning clinic: Absence of infection in an indigent population in San Francisco. *American Journal of Public Health, 79*(7), 883-885.

Downing, M., Knight, K., Vernon, K., Seigel, S., Ajaniku, I., Acosta, P., Thomas, L., and Porter, S. (1999). This is my story: A descriptive analysis of peer education HIV/STD risk reduction program for women living in public housing. *AIDS Education and Prevention, 11*(3), 243-261.

Oliva, G., Rienks, J., and McDermid, M. (1999). What high risk women are telling us about access to primary and reproduction health care and HIV prevention services. *AIDS Education and Prevention, 11*(6), 513-524.

Prochaska, J.O. and DiClemente, C.C. (1984). *The Transtheoretical Approach: Crossing the Traditional Boundaries of Therapy.* Homewood, IL: Dow-Jones/Irwin.

San Francisco Department of Public Health (SFDPH) (1990). HIV Seroprevalence Reports. *1,* 1-13.

Chapter 8

The Challenges and Rewards of Collaborative Research: The UFO Study

Kristen Ochoa
Rachel McLean
Heather Edney-Meschery
Dante Brimer
Andrew Moss

In memory of Dante Brimer, February 3, 1978—January 19, 2001

Teachers and students (leadership and people), co-intent on reality, are both subjects, not only in the task of unveiling reality, and thereby coming to know it critically, but in the task of recreating knowledge. As they attain this knowledge of reality through common reflection and action, they discover themselves as its permanent recreators. In this way, the presence of the oppressed in the struggle for their liberation will be what it should be: not pseudo-participation, but committed involvement.

Paulo Freire, *Pedagogy of the Oppressed* (1970)

A TYPICAL DAY IN THE UFO STUDY

At a punk show, Ivy bumps into Jeanie and Wolf and reminds them that their shots are due. In a San Francisco jail holding cell, while detained and awaiting release, Fur recruits other youths for HIV and hepatitis screening. At the study site, Ace stumbles in the door, short of breath. He is met by staff member Dante, another veteran of street life, who alerts other staffers that Ace is about to have a seizure. Elsewhere at the site, Kelly draws a study participant's blood and shows him a better vein to use for injections. The research director asks an outreach worker for advice; together, they rewrite a study question.

The "You Find-Out" (UFO) study, named by the young injectors it studies, brings together a diverse and interdisciplinary team of epidemiologists, outreach workers, physicians, interviewers, and counselors. Its goal is good science and good service, approached pragmatically. The community-based organization involves the researcher to further the agency's mission; the researcher involves the community-based organization to successfully complete the study. Both parties invite at-risk youth to become part of the planning and execution of the project.

INTRODUCTION

This chapter describes our experience with the UFO study, a collaborative research project involving service agencies and an academic research institution. Funded by the University-wide AIDS Research Program (UARP) of the state of California, the goal of the study was to document the prevalence of HIV, hepatitis B virus (HBV), and hepatitis C virus (HCV) infections among young injection-drug users in San Francisco and to better understand the factors that put youths at risk of infection. It was later expanded to reach drug-injecting youths in the city of Santa Cruz.

The ultimate goal of the project was to design lifesaving intervention programs. We hope that it may provide a useful approach to those faced with the complex challenge of combining the interests of researchers with those of community-based service providers.

DOING RESEARCH DIFFERENTLY

Many critics of traditional research, particularly in the public health field, are experimenting with a broader approach. Attempts have increased to create collaborative research between community-based organizations (CBOs) and academic institutions. In this model, the CBO staff, who understands the needs and concerns of the population being served, work with the researchers to identify important study questions—questions that define and illuminate the specific problems of the population. Together, the service providers and the researchers can attempt an intervention, then evaluate its success or failure. Using this approach, the success of research is measured not just by publication in professional journals, but by what happens during the process of the study.

Because it requires the involvement of the community, the collaborative approach is an exercise in participation for those being studied as well as those doing the studying. Collaborative research recognizes that study participants, as well as the organizations that serve them, have expertise—and thus seeks their involvement. Through such collaboration, participatory research can become participatory action—when the act of research creates change (Seal et al., 2000). Because it values the opinions of study participants, this strategy offers a more equal distribution of power than that which exists between researchers and community groups in the traditional approach. The two constituencies become coinvestigators; equally intent on gaining the knowledge they need to create social change.

The UFO study grew out of exploratory research with young injection drug users in San Francisco (Fernandes and Tandon, 1981), a continuation of the principal investigator's longtime interest in studies of HIV in injection drug users. Based on the exploratory research, a small, street-based, HIV prevalence study was funded with a grant from the Kaiser Family Foundation in 1996. A relationship between UCSF and the Haight-Ashbury Youth Outreach Team (HAYOT) of the Haight-Ashbury Free Clinics, Inc. (HAFCI) developed during this study and was formalized with two-year funding from the UARP in 1997. Once funded, we set out to look closely at HIV, hepatitis B (HBV), and hepatitis C (HCV) among young injectors in four neighborhoods of San Francisco.

For the UFO study team, participation by the study population was a natural extension of the principles of harm reduction. These principles were already accepted, to varying extents, by the researchers and the service providers. A basic tenet of harm reduction is the meaningful involvement of active and former drug users in the creation of programs designed to serve them (Harm Reduction Coalition, 1997). In applying this principle to our research, we employed young injection drug users as peer-outreach workers and peer-access interviewers in the study. In a London-based study, which used this approach, researchers reported that "privileged access interviewers" were key in the evaluation of harm reduction initiatives, and that peer interviewers were able to gain access to individuals not available to conventional research staff (Griffiths, 1993). For the academic staff of the UFO study, this particular finding was instrumental in providing a conceptual base from which to launch the project.

As AIDS activists and researchers, we also came to the table with an understanding of the history of the AIDS movement. Since the 1980s, AIDS activists and scientists have come together to combat the AIDS epidemic. As Steven Epstein writes, "the case of AIDS activism suggests that social movements can pursue distinctive forms of participation in science and, conversely, that the engagement with science can shape such movements in powerful ways" (1996, p. 382). With this recent historical precedent of collaboration, most of us believed at the outset of the study that we would benefit from one another's perspectives and experiences.

With input from service providers and study participants, the research project changed priorities over time. First, it became clear that HBV and, more particularly, HCV posed as great a threat as HIV to the drug-injecting population. Although we continued to test for HIV infections, we shifted our emphasis toward investigating hepatitis. Second, we observed that that needle exchange programs offered an opportunity to test new approaches to intervention. With a supplement to our UARP grant, we were able to extend the UFO project to the needle exchange program in Santa Cruz. Third, we realized the importance of vaccinating drug-injecting youths—first as a service responsibility, and then, when we recognized the difficulty of delivering HBV vaccines to young injectors, as a subsequent research project. Finally, when we realized that overdoses were the major cause of death in young injectors, we launched an investigation of ways to prevent drug overdose.

This shift in focus during the course of the study was the direct result of the close involvement of the researchers with the service providers and the young injectors themselves.

We continued this collaboration between the service providers, researchers, and clients while developing the study protocol and instrument. Because we would be testing hundreds of youths for HBV and HCV as well as HIV, we realized immediately that we had to create methods for hepatitis testing and counseling which would parallel the well-established testing and counseling approach for HIV. Moreover, we were faced with the ethical dilemma of disclosing negative serological status for HBV to a high-risk population without offering protective immunization.

The team went to the San Francisco Department of Public Health and received an ample supply of HBV vaccines. Then, with no research goal in mind, we began to offer the vaccinations to all participants who were not already immune. We enlisted the help of clinicians from the Tom Waddell Health Center of the city and county of San Francisco and the Haight-Ashbury Free Medical Clinic to provide vaccinations to study participants on site, then made appointments with the youths to return for follow-up booster shots. Finally, with a questionnaire, recruitment strategy, HBV vaccines, and a team of peer recruiters, interviewers, counselors, and medical providers in place, the study began. During busy times, we would see as many as twenty-five young people in one evening, and our sites started becoming big drop-in centers—places where we were able to do much more than research.

Various lengthy and unmemorable names were suggested for the study. One night at a study site, we asked the study participants to come up with something better. A young woman, thinking about her test results, suggested "U-Find Out." Our medical director, delighted by the idea that flying saucer symbols would help youths to remember when their shots were due, ran to the store and bought alien toys, spaceship stickers, and extraterrestrial party hats for the study site. Soon all the outreach materials featured UFOs and we and the young injectors both started referring to the project as the "UFO study."

THE STUDY

During its work from 1997 to 1999 the UFO study interviewed 696 injection drug users under the age of thirty years. A preliminary analysis found that the average age of participants was twenty-two years old. They had been injecting drugs, on average, for five years. Although the vast majority had participated in needle exchange programs an average of three years, 46 percent reported borrowing a used syringe within the past year.

The study found that almost one-half of the youths were infected with HCV, one-third were infected with HBV, and 6 percent with HIV. Only 13 percent of the youths had evidence of vaccination against HBV.

The study gained a second objective: delivering hepatitis B vaccination to these young injectors. In a pilot vaccine study, 183 of 228, or 80 percent, of eligible study participants received the first vaccine.

The most common reason for lack of vaccination was failure of youths to return for test results—a fact that reflects the transience of the population. But with an incentive payment of $10 to those who returned for their second and third vaccine doses, two-thirds received their second dose and one-half received their third dose.

We found that overdosing was the most immediate health concern among young injection-drug users. Among 312 youths studied, 55 percent reported at least one overdose and 75 percent had witnessed an overdose. When witnessing a drug overdose, 52 percent said they had called 911, 61 percent performed CPR, and 72 percent kept the person awake by walking him or her around or shaking him or her. Eleven percent reported that the injector had died.

We invited outreach workers from agencies in the four surrounding neighborhoods to meet the participants and provide referrals for long-term follow-up. The vaccine intervention project evolved into a follow-up study to explore how to best deliver the HBV vaccine to this difficult-to-reach population. As the blood-testing phase of the study came to an end, and vaccine issues became more important, we concentrated on two study sites, one in the Haight-Ashbury area and one in the Mission District.

In an effort to bring testing, counseling, and vaccination into a needle exchange setting, we set out to provide "technology transfer" to the Santa Cruz Needle Exchange, creating "UFO Santa Cruz." Santa Cruz was chosen as a collaborator for several reasons. The San Francisco Needle Exchange at that time was not receptive to incorporating this kind of research into its needle exchange activities. Second, San Francisco's traditional needle exchange programs attract an older crowd of drug users. Santa Cruz not only had experience working with researchers, they previously had been involved in another UARP collaboration. In addition, the Santa Cruz Needle Exchange is known for its ability to attract and serve young injection-drug users. This small but well-organized needle exchange program seemed like the ideal place for us to recreate UFO.

The project has been a success. But it has not been without its challenges. With so many different people involved, everyone has developed their own perspective as to which aspects of the project have worked well—and which have been more difficult.

In the spirit of participation, the UFO team describes their perspectives in their own voices, so that the reader may directly observe how our approaches, ambitions, misfortunes, and successes converge and diverge.

BEGINNING IN THE MIDDLE

In Paul Farmer's book, *Infections and Inequalities,* he describes how his work with the peasants of Haiti began. He asks a local priest about conducting a formal needs assessment. "Fine," the priest tells him, "but they're just going to tell you they want a hospital." When the needs assessment is over, Farmer explains that the priest was correct; most people surveyed wanted a hospital. Then, he writes, "Notably, we never heard requests for research" (Farmer, 1999, p. 19).

The sentiment among the underserved that research is unimportant in a resource-poor environment seems almost universal. Trade the shacks of the village for the doorways of the city, add heroin, speed, and crack, and you get the same basic needs: shelter, food, medical care, and treatment. No one living in the street cares much about research. The job of the researcher, then, becomes one of justifying his or her presence or minimizing its impact. When I (Kristen Ochoa) came to the Department of Epidemiology, research into the emerging population of young injection-drug users was inevitable. Investigators around the country, and within our own institution, were vying for a piece of the young injector "turf." I joined in the study of young injectors somewhat cautiously, but I did so believing that we could equally provide both data and service for this very vulnerable population.

The UFO study started with a call from Marc Sabin, who directed the Haight-Ashbury Youth Outreach Team. He came across a request for proposals from the University-wide AIDS Research Program and described the application to me over the phone. It was ideal, and I immediately began to think of it as a joint service and research endeavor. It was one project with two goals—the best of both worlds. As it turned out, the grant was written more with research in mind than service, so it became a major challenge, once we were funded, to establish a project that was going to produce more than just study findings.

The Tensions

The idea was not merely to design compelling research that would protect or improve the health of young injectors in the future—but to create a research environment where we could help them from the moment that we first met them.

We did succeed in providing testing and counseling, vaccinations, outreach, food, and basic medical care to all of those we surveyed, and this was made easier by the collaboration. The research staff and the youth outreach staff truly had different priorities, but we were fortunate to have a team of open minds. Our weekly meetings were often contentious, but we constantly negotiated. For instance, epidemiologists had a different concept than the outreach workers of what it meant to work with the youths. On such occasions, the service staff spoke up, often supported by myself and by the study medical director Paula Lum. As a physician, Lum straddled the fence between science and patient care. All of these disagreements and differences were heard and considered, regardless of the outcome. We all knew that if something wasn't going well, we just needed to bring it to the table.

Though we have moved in the direction of participatory research, we have not yet arrived at complete participation. Even though our team was comprised of many members, principal investigator Andrew Moss always made the final decisions. It would be difficult to find an investigator so open and willing to be involved in this collaboration. Moss came to almost every site, just to be there and talk with staff and study participants. Everyone knew him. He acted democratically and did not make decisions without input. Still, research is never entirely participatory until the community representatives have equal decision-making power. This said, I consider the work of UFO to be a giant leap in the right direction.

In an earlier pilot of the study, several peer interviewers were hired who were very successful at going out on the street and surveying people at needle exchanges and other venues. One of the youngest and most well liked peer workers went home from work one night and overdosed in her apartment. By the time the fire department arrived, it was too late. She was so well known in harm reduction circles that the whole movement seemed to stand still for the time following her overdose. We took pause and considered what we were doing: HIV prevention *and* hepatitis research seemed off the mark. Why were we focusing on infection when our friends were dying—not of AIDS, not of hepatitis—but of overdose?

Being Responsive

Priorities changed. We had to find out why youths were dying of overdose. Without any formal funding, and without any precedent in the United States to do this kind of study, we began to form focus groups to ask people what they thought was happening. I engaged the help of two young drug injectors who did secondary exchange (exchanged needles for others) from their hotel room. Oreo and Fur knew a lot of young people on the street and in single-resident-occupancy hotels who were young injection-drug users. They became our link. The staff would set up the field site, and Oreo and Fur would bring in ten, twenty, sometimes forty different kids. They came to research meetings, and both were eventually put on the payroll. The UFO study could not have worked without Oreo and Fur.

By working alongside interviewers and counselors who have academic and professional backgrounds, the peers allowed us to do the job right. It takes special care and attention to manage such a multidisciplinary team, but it is well worth the effort since the team is constantly learning from one another. This is why our study has been so successful and so popular with the youths. The kids really like coming to see us; sometimes they come just to say hello. We have good adherence to the hepatitis B vaccine regimen, no doubt, because our outreach workers truly know our participants. In terms of legitimacy, it is rare that we enroll someone who is not young and not injecting because our screening system is so good.

Having a middleman (or middle woman, as it were) is important in collaboration. All collaborations need a marriage counselor—someone who can't take sides and whose job it is to help partners communicate. All collaborations need someone whose job it is to get people invested in the project through communication. Someone should be appointed just to make sure that everyone believes that they have a voice, that they are learning, and that they are productive.

As an employee of the research institution, but as an ally and former staffer with the Haight-Ashbury Free Clinics, Inc., I was in a unique position to see both sides. It was not easy, however. I spent many hours listening to concerns and trying to represent the position of others, while defending my own position or not taking any position at all. Most of the pressure to take sides came from the research staff. Once, they told me I was "pitting the field staff against the researchers." However, the field staff also criticized me, asking "how can you let them make us ask these study questions?" It was difficult to not take a position, or to take both positions (i.e., as researcher and provider) and to see both sides equally, but it seemed to serve the study well to have a go-between who could move in and out of both worlds. In time, everyone on staff got better at seeing both sides and the opposition gradually faded.

Youth-Centered Project

In the end, it really all comes down to the participants—the youths. They made the study possible and they are affected most by the success or failure of the collaborative. If the project is a disaster, they pay the price by being treated apathetically or by answering questionnaires that never get analyzed. If the study flourishes, they benefit from immediate attention to their individual needs; and as a population, they benefit from research that will affect the broader health policy agenda in their favor.

This study lasted only two years, but we are already seeing its impact. The youths have been influenced by the research; and they have influenced the research. Many participants have told us that before we came, no one knew what hepatitis was, and no one had been tested for it. Nor had they thought much about overdose prevention. Now that the information is everywhere, there is constant talk of the risks. The UFO research staff also changed. Each staff member came face-to-face with the problem he or she was studying. Before the UFO study, a research staff member said, "I could never do this, it's so intense." But she has now done it with UFO. Over time, in fact, all of the research staff became very involved in the fieldwork. The UFO project has changed the culture of the UCSF Department of Epidemiology and Biostatistics, transforming its mission from conducting passive to active research.

The phenomenon of UFO can be named in many ways: collaboration, harm reduction, participatory action research, anarchy, punk, communism, or common sense. True collaborative research is a kind of alchemy. For the researcher, it is watching data come to life. Even if the papers are not published, even if no more abstracts are accepted to conferences, we still vaccinated 362 people, tested and counseled 717 people for HIV and hepatitis B and C, and gave a handful of youths pride in their work and showed hundreds of others that we cared about them.

THE COMMUNITY COLLABORATOR'S PERSPECTIVE

On the street and in the world, outside of academia, a lot of people are wary of research, and with good reason. It's easy for researchers to just pick one aspect of people's lives that they find most interesting, and to ignore the rest. Yet, this prioritization is often in contradiction to what the people know are their most pressing needs. By having such a narrow focus, researchers dismiss the complex realities of the people they propose to study and miss the details that could really teach them something new.

The Haight-Ashbury Youth Outreach Team (HAYOT) collaboration with UCSF began with a brief pilot study in which we found out that the young injectors we work with knew little about hepatitis B. They were at high risk, yet few had ever been vaccinated. The UARP grant presented an ideal opportunity for shedding additional light on the issues of HIV and hepatitis, as well as securing funding for our outreach activities, providing documentation of the health status of our population, and providing an evaluation of our program. We ended up gaining all of these things, and a whole lot more.

Early into the UFO study we were shocked to discover that while few of our clients had HIV, half of them (average age twenty-two) were testing positive for hepatitis C. Project staff also found that the young injectors were overdosing, their friends were overdosing, and they did not know what to do. Prior to this, funding and outreach priorities were dominated by HIV prevention. The findings of the UFO study led to a dramatic shift in prevention activities and priorities. Prevention messages moved from HIV: "bleach for thirty seconds," to HIV *and* hepatitis C messages: "always use new cookers, cottons, rigs, and equipment." Now the focus is on overdose prevention much more heavily in our outreach, and are working with the San Francisco Department of Public Health's Treatment on Demand Planning Council to finalize recommendations around hepatitis C and overdose awareness and prevention. In the three-and one-half years that I (Rachel McLean) have been working here, I have seen over a dozen youth die of heroin overdose. Yet the UFO study is the only research project in this country focusing on this issue, and one of the first to focus on hepatitis C. I am proud to have been part of this collaborative. Ironically enough, it took working with outside researchers to get us to get our priorities right!

Health Benefits

Standing in the phlebotomy room (slash office, slash storage space for socks and snacks) with Dr. Paula Lum of the UFO study, I'm thinking to myself, *"Damn, this is pretty cool."* Look at all the stuff we're doing for the kids. Here we are in our shabby/funky Youth Outreach office getting the kids tested for HIV, hepatitis B, and hepatitis C. Not only that, but we're giving them free vaccine, paying them and chasing them across the whole continent to remind them to get their follow-up shots. This is something maybe a few kids would do on their own, but even the free clinic doesn't even have access to unlimited free vaccines. Even if they did, kids would rarely follow up, being as transient as they are. Yet here we are in this space that the Haight-Ashbury Youth Outreach Team has made safe after six years of trust-building and hard work, providing services governed by the needs of the youth.

Since the beginning of HAYOT's work with UCSF, the level of awareness raising among the young injectors in the Haight-Ashbury area and throughout the city has been incredible. Constantly, youths share information with one another about their hepatitis C status, how to prevent it, and how to get tested. More new users know to ask for cookers and cottons every time they use. They police their friends about sharing equipment. They explain to one another the importance of getting vaccinated and the meaning of a liver function test. In fact, friends refer most participants to UFO. When asked why they return for vaccinations, some users reply, "Just knowing that I'm taking care of myself."

In the process of finding out their HIV and hepatitis status and getting vaccinated, young people are taking small steps to take care of themselves, and one another. Having the testing and vaccinations take place at HAYOUT's outreach office enables follow-up with liver function tests, information on self-care for people with hepatitis C, and most important, follow-up hepatitis A and B vaccine. It has also introduced a lot of young indoor and hotel-dwelling injectors to the services. This is the true meaning of a win-win situation between community-based work and research.

Enhanced Quality of Research Atmosphere

My job, with the help of my fellow outreach workers Ivy and Ben, has been to play hostess, hand out supplies, and deal with as many peoples' needs as I can. Often, at least one of us already knows the participant, but if we don't, we make sure to establish a relationship on the spot. Often, that means setting up a time to meet them again, inviting them to come back anytime, or telling them about services such as food, showers, and free pet-care vouchers. In this way, the seeds of long-term trust are planted so that, later on, when people have other questions or have friends that have questions, they know where to find us. With medics on site, we talk about abscesses, vein care, drug detox, and whatever other issues are relevant. Time passes and participants come back, wanting to work for us, because we treated them with respect. Or they draw us pictures of the Virgin of Guadalupe surrounded by UFOs and send them to us from jail. This is long-lasting friendship.

When people bring in their friends and partners that means they are talking about things—about their status, about sharing rigs and equipment, about having unprotected sex. The seeds of contemplation and change have been planted. They know they can come back anytime. That seed gets watered a little bit more every time. A week later it's a quick question, and a month later it's help getting into detox, or a resume, or "Will you come with me to get my liver function test?" or "When can I start working for you guys?"

Validation and Self-Esteem for Youth

The UFO study has allowed users to step into the light and feel the validation of someone official paying attention to their health needs and offering real assistance. In turn, HAYOUT has served as a cultural competency and peer-access bridge for UCSF to reach the hard-core users, those most at risk for hepatitis C and overdose who are not being reached by other service providers. When the staff respects participants, they see an opportunity to change their lives. Michelle, a young woman/participant/volunteer, was talking about a job she applied for. She felt she was being watched and treated more cautiously because of her drug use. She said, "I thought it was like the UFO study. I thought I could be honest and tell them I was using. I didn't want to have to lie." Perhaps it was a misleading message for someone who was joining the mainstream workforce, but she knew she could be herself with us, and that we would accept her no matter what.

Working outside the Haight, strengthening interagency ties, conducting outreach into other neighborhoods, and reminding participants to get their follow-up shots enables HAYOUT to follow up with the clients who have not been seen in a while and offer hope to those too "tore back" to even ask for help. While doing outreach in the Castro, my co-worker and I ran into Kali who had just gotten out of jail and was having a hard time. She asked about the UFO study and said that she wanted to do it the whole time she was in jail. She told us she had hepatitis C and was worried about it. We told her to get vaccinated against hepatitis A and B, so that she did not get any extra liver damage.

Long after the UFO study is gone, the HAYOT will be here, maintaining that relationship. Conducting outreach throughout the city has also enabled HAYOUT to collaborate with other agencies doing outreach in other neighborhoods. For youths that live and hang out in other neighborhoods, HAYOUT ensures that they connect with trustworthy local outreach workers who can establish ongoing relationships as well.

Agency Legitimacy and a Positive Evaluation

As an agency, HAYOT is committed to working with the kids no one else wants to serve. Our dedication to the most hard-core users and our harm-reduction approach sometimes alienates us both from local residents, merchants, other service providers, and the powers that be. Working with UCSF has been good in terms of legitimizing our work, as well as the youths we work with. In addition, the evaluation results of the hepatitis B vaccination outreach showed that our efforts increased adherence by 64 percent.

For outreach workers, having the opportunity to codetermine the priorities of the research agenda has been a refreshing change from the top-down approach of most research and policy settings. Throughout the collaboration, outreach workers' opinions were highly valued amidst medical doctors, epidemiologists, ethnographers, and PhDs. I have been consistently asked,

> Rachel, we're just stuffy academics. Tell us, what do you think? You're the expert. Tell us what the reality is. Will this idea work with these kids? What's going on around Haight Street? What's going on with the neighbors and the cops? What are the kids' needs *and* what should we be doing differently?

Paulo Freire's concept of participatory research has definitely been put into practice in this project. Throughout the collaboration we were given implicit permission to speak our minds.

Input from the staff helps and all of this makes for a lively debate on any decision. Participants have become outreach workers, and HAYOT clients have become interviewers . . . all the kids want to work for the study because it's "cool." All along the way there has been an understanding that it is important to ask the kids and the staff their thoughts about how to solve a problem. It hasn't always been easy—but we've worked things out and I feel proud to be a part of the UFO Team.

Difficulties

Strain on Already Limited Resources

The level of integration between HAYOT and UCSF was both the strength and the weakness of the collaboration (see Box 8.1). When the project began, the UARP grant was one of numerous funding sources for five outreach workers. Over the course of the study, our director, Marc Sabin resigned, leaving us with no fund-raiser and

BOX 8.1. The Advantages and Disadvantages of Collaborative Research: The Community Perspective

PROS

Practical support: Expenses (staff, rent, supplies) paid by research.

Health benefits for the youths: Increased awareness and agency, HIV, Hepatitis B and C Testing. Free hepatitis A and B vaccines and medical attention.

Validation and self-esteem for youths: Calls attention to the health needs of the population. Increased self-worth for participants. Potential for hire as peer educators creates tangible incentive for change.

Enhanced quality of research atmosphere: Cultural competency makes better research and happier participants.

Community building and strengthening ties with other agencies: Doing outreach in other neighborhoods creates a good opportunity for community building and collaboration with other CBOs, as well as influential researchers.

Agency legitimacy and a positive evaluation: CBO legitimized, relationships with neighborhood, government and other agencies improve. Provides documentation of efficacy of outreach and collaboration.

A voice in research and a good relationship: Keeps research responsible/responsive to the needs of the community. Provides community access to research and policymaking agendas. Creates a long-standing relationship to build on in the future.

CONS

Strain on already limited resources: Time and resource commitment. Degree of strain on community agency depends on levels of staffing, proportion of total staff time/resources devoted to project. Financial strain on agency when check comes later than proposed start-up date.

Conflicts of interest between research and service provision: It is difficult turning participants away. May jeopardize street credibility. Also, research and service aims blur.

Conflicts around cultural competency between researchers, providers, and participants: "Academic speak" intimidating for community providers. Research staff may not understand culture of population.

Shifts outreach/services focus to fit the research agenda: Sets outreach agenda, shifts resources away from agency's regular focus. Sets tone away from being client-centered. Outreach workers may feel their access to the population is being exploited.

Ethical issues, such as the lack of social support, testing, and changes in the power dynamic: It is difficult to ask depression/social support questions. Inability to meet broad range of needs in quick outreach sessions after results disclosure. Not as easy in neighborhoods other than your own.

Increases visibility of services: Strain on building. May be disastrous depending on degree of neighborhood opposition to services only two grants between three remaining outreach workers. This was circumstantial, and by no means the fault of our research collaborators. If anything, this study saved our agency from sinking completely. But having two out of three staff members dedicate half their time to this project put a strain on our daily drop-in, outreach, and administrative operations, which at that time were performed by the outreach workers. Some staff felt stretched thin by dual roles.

Conflicts of Interest Between Research and Service Provision

At times, a conflict of interest arose between the research and service agendas. It has been hard to turn away kids that don't qualify for the study. They inevitably say, "just lie for me!" We worked for years to establish a relationship with them. Loyalties were divided between the kids and research protocol. This felt very difficult at first but got easier with time, especially as kids knew what to expect. Having an ongoing relationship with people—and making sure that anyone we had to turn away left with their hands full of free food, sodas, supplies, bus tokens, socks, or referrals—helped a lot.

The line between service provision and research often became a point of contention in research staff meetings when conflicts of interest arose. There is a tendency to want to do it all, but we also know from experience that when research endeavors attempt to duplicate services, the results can be disastrous when funding ends and the community is left reeling from a program's absence. In instances such as this be clear about your intentions. Are you just doing this to make yourself feel better, or are you doing this because it actually makes sense and is what people want? Research should inform services, not duplicate them—but what if nobody's doing them at all? This was the case with hepatitis testing and vaccination. If necessary, do it first as research, then ask for support to keep it going on its own accord.

Conflicts Regarding Cultural Competency

Conflicts also arose regarding cultural competency, both between collaborators, and between clients and staff. The outreach staff was initially intimidated by the academic jargon used by researchers.

Even after I learned how to decipher the jargon, I saw new outreach staff feeling equally intimidated and not necessarily faring as well in deciphering this cryptic language of significance and probability. Overall, we fared amazingly well but frustrations exploded on several occasions when either researchers or community-based staff felt disrespected. At the UFO sites, some tense moments arose when staff, who were not used to dealing with street youths, overstepped boundaries that they didn't even know were there. Outreach workers were usually around to intervene, but sometimes they got caught in the middle.

Shifts of Outreach/Services Focus to Fit Research Agenda

When HAYOUT began the UFO study, along with the HIV and hepatitis testing, it offered youths free vaccinations and telling participants to come back for free follow-up shots. UFO-2 began as a way to improve adherence—to prove that this population could be vaccinated. But this soon turned into the sole focus of outreach. Originally, focus had been on recruiting and playing "outreach hostess" at the UFO sites. Recruiting was a cinch and happened mostly through word of mouth. UFO outreach became a separate entity from HAYOT outreach because it involved a heavy focus on other neighborhoods, phone calls, postcards, and a perpetual "wild-goose chase." This became very exhausting and a strain on the agency, which at that point, consisted only of two people.

These efforts would have been feasible with a larger staff or a more stable group. Running around and tracking people down for hepatitis B vaccinations was not the intent of the collaboration.

Ethical Issues

Ethical issues also came up. We were testing and reminding people whose lives were miserable to get their shots. We were fragmenting kids' lives like all the rest—some aspects of that are inevitable. If the kids had complete decision-making power, it wouldn't have been like that.

It's hard giving positive HIV and hepatitis C results when the resources are so limited and when people's lives and psyches are already taxed. We tell people to come back for their results when they're ready, but there is still that anxiety of "what if they didn't really want to know?" This all goes back to the reluctance some have about testing people for HIV and hepatitis and then following them across the country to remind them to get vaccinated, when they "haven't got a pot to piss in." Food, drugs, money, and shelter always come first before health. Those bases may never be covered adequately, however, the multitude of issues young injectors face must be acknowledged.

This dilemma came up for outreach workers in UFO-2 study. It's sad not being able to make people's lives much better, just reminding them that there's someone out there that cares. But it's more than that. It's this sick feeling I got in my stomach a while back when I was on 16th and Mission Streets and ran into a couple of the participants that we've been trying to find for a while.

"Hey, what are you guys up to?" I ask.

"Just trying to make money," one says.

I know, by the way they rush-walk, asking is just a formality. I hesitate because they're crossing the street and don't want to deal with what I represent. Yet I've been looking for them all this time. Usually I would let them set the terms of the conversation. But being an outreach worker for the research study means that I come into this situation with an agenda. I want to say that I got them to come in for their shots because that's a big part of my job and I want to be doing it well. But I feel like I'm crossing the line in some way. They don't want a "reality check" right now. Even though it's for their benefit, I'm the one setting the priorities. Like, "Hey, I know you're dope-sick and just got kicked out of your hotel and you're totally miserable, but did you know you're due for your shot?"

All they say is, "We know, we know." Which just confirms my belief that they have more immediate needs to deal with right now, which is why they haven't come in. I'm sure there's an element of shame, too, of having us see them going so far downhill. As much as we're trying to reach people on their level, there's still that element of power in the dynamics, suggested in these words:

indoor	homeless
researcher	subject
outreach worker	client
fed	hungry
rested	exhausted

clean-clothed	unclean clothes
showered	"dirty/smelly"
employed	drug dealer/hustler
nonuser, or user	stigmatized "junkie"

There is this unwritten law: as an outreach worker, you develop trust slowly over a long period of time. You check in to see how people are doing and sometimes they want to deal with big life questions, and sometimes they just want to talk about the little things. You work together—but they set the terms. The difficulty of doing outreach for research lies in this subtle difference: No matter how compassionate you are, you are still there with an agenda, and it shows.

In the end, the culmination of these dynamics led us to end our collaboration with UCSF. The time and resource constraints as well as the way that the collaboration shifted our outreach agenda away from our primary focus of supporting homeless youths in the Haight became too much. In July 1999, an expected grant fell through, funding evaporated, and HAYOT went with it. Facing an eviction from our space, we decided to end the collaboration in order to save what was left of our program. We have since recovered, although in reduced form. I have only positive feelings for the UFO study. We will continue to support it. I have learned a tremendous amount from this collaboration, and maintain the utmost love and respect for the UFO staff, who, by the way, rule the world.

THE SANTA CRUZ NEEDLE EXCHANGE

We knew about the UFO Study long before it came to Santa Cruz. Kristen Ochoa and I (Heather Edney-Meschery), both long-time needle exchange organizers, knew and trusted one another through years of working together. Though our program was eager to find out how to do relevant hepatitis prevention, our first attempts at creating educational materials weren't effective. We were rarely able to engage our program participants in conversations about hepatitis that were meaningful to their daily lives. When we were asked if we would be interested in collaborating with UCSF, we were not only given the opportunity to interview participants, test them and vaccinate them, but we were also given a chance to engage them about their risk for hepatitis, something we could not do before.

During the course of a person's participation in the UFO study, he or she had the opportunity to interact with several different staff members. At the front desk, staff explained the criteria for the study and answered initial questions about hepatitis. While waiting to get their blood drawn, participants were served hot food and could hang out with volunteers trained to answer questions about the study and hepatitis transmission. Participants came in for the interview, where they had a chance to talk about sharing their works, overdose, and other issues. As they left, they were offered literature on hepatitis prevention that we designed specifically for the group of kids in the study. When the kids came back for their test results and vaccination, they met with the same staff members and had another opportunity to ask questions and talk about their concerns. Throughout the course of their participation in the UFO study, there were many opportunities for intervention and many chances for the participants to get the information and care that they needed.

At the drop-in center, we provide literature—and like all drop-in centers, we have a lot of literature. Because it looked more interesting than the more mainstream flyers on hepatitis, people were more apt to pick it up and check it out. They generally asked about the study, which opened a conversation about hepatitis prevention. Also, participants would see the UFO posters and ask "What does UFO stand for?" or "What does that mean?" which gave the staff and volunteers an entrée for discussion.

In addition to all of the prevention opportunities with our participants, the UFO study legitimized needle exchange in the eyes of the Santa Cruz County Health Department in a way that we had not experienced previously. The Department of Communicable Diseases at the Santa Cruz Health Services Agency was totally uninvolved with the needle exchange, even though we had been doing HIV prevention for over ten years in Santa Cruz County. But when we began collaborating with UCSF, the department began to show an interest in us, visiting the drop-in site and offering support. Later, they approached us about writing a collaborative grant to continue the UFO programming with us. For the first time, they proposed to write a grant with us not because they needed access to our population, but because they needed access to our expertise. Recently, they notified us that they will support the project on an ongoing basis. Hopefully, this new relationship with the health department will result in greater protection of the needle exchange program. As they become more invested in our interventions, they may ultimately become reliant upon our program staying open.

Another profound impact of the UFO/Santa Cruz collaboration has been that the staff, volunteers, and participants don't just talk about HIV anymore. The whole purpose of the drop-in center has shifted focus to include hepatitis, simply because that is what is affecting the greatest number of people.

UFO has also given us the opportunity to publish another edition of *Junkphood,* our zine created by and for injection drug users, now on its eighth volume. Participants talk about their own experiences—saying what it's like to get a positive hepatitis result, what it means to them to get vaccinated, and how they can avoid infections in the future. It also includes the outcome of the study and the rates of hepatitis B, C, HIV, and overdose in a way that is easy to read and understand. Because *Junkphood* is distributed nationally, we know that the UFO edition will reach many people far beyond Santa Cruz. As a result of a recent feature on overdose, the Lindesmith Center (a George Soros-funded foundation) purchased a large number of zines to distribute at their first International Conference on Preventing Heroin Overdose in Seattle.

The UFO study, however, has not come without its disadvantages. There is no way we could ever have been prepared, either programmatically or emotionally, to give so many positive results to so many people. The greatest challenge has been helping them strategize about how they can get help in a county with so few resources.

Also frustrating is the fact that the UFO Study only involved injectors under thirty years of age. Drug injectors of all ages come to us, and none have adequate access to health care. To deny older injectors something that we know they need is bad public health. People over twenty-nine should know their status and be offered a vaccine. Until the county steps up to help with our efforts, this will continue to be a frustration and limitation that we have to deal with. At one point we only had funding for four more tests and there was a possibility that the study would be ending. One week later, the department of public health informed Santa Cruz Needle Exchange that it wanted us to continue the testing and vaccinations for people of all ages. If we had not had the support of UCSF in making this study happen, these services would not be available to injectors in Santa Cruz.

Overall, the UFO study has given Santa Cruz Needle Exchange the opportunity to continue to interact with the youths in our program with whom we already have good relationships. UFO is relevant to them. It's tangible. Even if the $10 incentive is what gets them in the door, they wind up getting such a high quality of care that the importance of the financial incentive diminishes.

For a brief time, our funding situation with UFO was at risk when UCSF did not receive the federal grant they expected. During this time, I received a letter from a participant who was in jail. He wrote: "I'm sorry to hear that the UFO study is running out of money. I think the study is one of the best I've ever seen. You're all doing great work at the DIC [drop-in center] and I can't wait to be a part of that group again."

THE PEER INTERVIEWER/COUNSELOR PERSPECTIVE

I (Dante Brimer) have been working at the UFO study in San Francisco for about a year now and I have seen its ups and its downs, but I have always believed in it because I have seen it do things that people with more money could not.

At its best, the UFO study is a well-oiled vaccinating, testing, harm-reducing, data-collecting machine. At its worst, it has not been a well-oiled, vaccinating, harm-reducing machine, staffed by a skeleton crew of volunteers who love the study and what it's about. It is harder when other epidemiologists try and take over, but it still works. The funding fiasco that temporarily disbanded the study was very heartbreaking. It broke up a team that got the job done—and got along well while doing it.

I am a former heroin addict and a former client of the Haight-Ashbury Youth Outreach Team. When I was about four months clean and sober, I started volunteering at the HAYOT. My first interviews were hard because I was so newly out of that life. But when it was difficult, there were always people to help me through it.

During the course of my work, I witnessed a very good team of people do a lot of good work.* Being able to relate to the participants has been a great tool in my harm-reduction counseling with them.

---

*Staff of the largest, most well-funded youth agency in San Francisco wear purple jackets while doing street outreach.

When I share some of my personal experiences with them, relating to them on a peer level, they usually respond well. My experiences also help in the collection of good data. Some kids would say that they were injectors when they really weren't, due to the free testing and $10 incentive. So to combat that problem, I was put in charge of screening the participants, armed with only a short questionnaire and my drug-use expertise. We were able to weed out almost all of the noninjectors.

I wish that we could test and vaccinate all of the people who walk through the door but we cannot. Sometimes my past experiences make my job more difficult. For instance, I have had to turn down interviews because I knew the person. I also had a person that I used to share needles with come in and test positive for hepatitis C.

We have seen a lot of kids complete their hepatitis B vaccinations, and we have seen kids get health care that they normally wouldn't have received without us. But one of the best parts of this job is when participants are excited to see you because they want to tell you about the positive changes they have made in their lives. When participants see where I have been able to go with my life, they know it is possible for them, too. I sure hope that we can get funding to do this for as long as there is a need for HIV and hepatitis testing.

THE RESEARCHER'S PERSPECTIVE

Walter Benjamin described the angel of history as looking backward, hurled rearward into the future by storms out of paradise and seeing history itself as the wreckage piled up at history's feet. I (Andrew Moss) think the angel of research faces backward too. She doesn't know where she's going because she's being blasted backward into the future by the winds out of the funding agencies. What she sees piled up around her feet are the papers the researchers somehow managed to write along the way.

Research studies are like little boats bobbing up and down in those storms that blow out of the funding agencies. The funding storms that bounce researchers up and down are only the biggest peril of the research business: there are also the political storms, the ethical storms, the turf-competition storms, and the personal storms. We push the boat out, the wind goes up and the storm rises, and if we're lucky we get back into harbor again with a useful result.

The high incidence of HBV and HCV in the young injector population was a surprise, since these injectors usually use clean needles. It was a useful stimulus to figure out why rates were so high, and what to do about intervention. Publication of this finding and the need for intervention was probably in itself a sufficient justification for the UARP study.

Another justification was the development of an intervention strategy for HBV vaccination. This was not part of the design of the UFO study. It evolved along the way due to community pressure to provide the vaccine to our study participants, once we discovered that very few of them had had it. The staff of HAYOUT started another study called the UFO 2 study—another little boat bobbing about in the storm—to seek ways to deliver HBV vaccination to young injectors. This has since become a principal agenda in the next stage of research. Getting these issues on the table was probably worth the money for the UARP.

Midway through the UARP study—in a process that beautifully demonstrates the semirandom workings of the funding process—we got a surprise supplement to our grant that enabled us to begin our collaboration with the Santa Cruz Needle Exchange. This allowed us to export both testing and vaccination to the needle exchange setting. The Santa Cruz exchange is one of the first groups in the country to do this. It may be the most important thing the UFO study accomplished; it was a major success of the project.

Along the way, we found that young injectors were overdosing, on average, once every two years. So the overdose issue became another major new research initiative. Overdose death is a real and present threat in the drug injector's world, something that even an academic researcher cannot ignore. This was the fourth major success of the study, one that wasn't even hinted at in the original proposal. Like the HBV vaccine study and the needle exchange intervention, the overdose issue came about because the community-collaborative side of the project put pressure on the academic researchers to design intervention strategies, rather than just testing people as the original grant proposed. Without UARP funding, UCSF researchers would not have studied this issue. It was the nature of the collaboration that put us "under the gun." This broadening of our scope, this redefinition of our research, took us away from the original serological goals funded by the UARP. The process of doing the study changed our priorities.

So, how should we rate the success of the study? First, in terms of our original serological goals, we found out a lot about HIV and hepatitis infection and presented it at many conferences and in quite a few publications. Second, our overdose data are the first to be generated from an American study. Third, we responded to pressure from the community to define important issues and interventions and got some of them put on the policy agenda. Fourth, we were awarded federal funding for the next phase of the UFO study, promoting it to the national level. Fifth, and perhaps the most rewarding outcome, the collaboration has been a success at the interpersonal level. We actually managed to keep the study afloat while engaging in academic-community interaction.

The community collaboration process worked because it dissolved the barriers between "us," the researchers, and "them," the subjects of our research. The community collaboration offered us a vital intermediary between the subjects and ourselves. It offered a means to probe into their lives, while buffering us from the psychic wounds of working with this very high-risk, very self-destructive, young population. These were immense benefits. We probably could not have done this study except as a community collaboration. However, there is a price for this, and the price was learning to live with culture clash.

Community collaboration can add a heavy burden to the load on research studies, due to the culture clash between researchers and activists. Culture clash is particularly evident in studies of drug users. The staffs of CBOs are invariably advocates for the "harm reduction" side of social polarization. They identify with the "kids." They are part of the rebel culture. They have attitude; they are politically correct. There is no way around all this. This is the nature of community collaboration.

A mark of true intelligence is the ability to keep two contradictory ideas in your head at the same time and keep functioning. Anyone doing community collaboration will need this type of intelligence, because there is a contradiction between the goals of the parties in the collaboration.

The goal of activists (which is what the community collaborators are) is to make life better for their clients. They think, correctly, that there is not always a direct link between what researchers discover and improvements in their clients' lives. They don't particularly trust academic investigators. They are right not to. They are right to defend their interests and the interests of their clients. We, the academics, tend not to be respectful of community turf. We probably don't understand the realities of life for young injectors.

Researchers, in contrast, tend to be concerned with publishing and the priorities of professional hierarchy. We would like to help people and have an interesting time, but these issues are sometimes secondary. When it comes to working with an "outsider" population like young injectors, we need collaborators to keep us honest. To do so, we must accept their priorities as having equal value with our own. Such acceptance may require some speedy tacking from the "principal investigator" at the helm. It definitely requires intelligence when the principal investigator has to recognize that behind the attitude, the "cult of the victims," and the political correctness, twenty-something-year-old community collaborators are actually *right*. It's an education. The culture clash has been both the upside and the downside of the UFO collaboration. However, it was immensely valuable.

The study was taken to the federal level, where the boats are bigger and events move more slowly. Things did not go smoothly. A hitch in funding the study, even though it had a reasonable priority score, left us out of funds for six months. The volatility of the funding process has been harder for community collaborators than for us.

What did we give the community collaborators? The answer may be a certain kind of legitimacy, perhaps. Perhaps they got some publicity that they wouldn't have had otherwise, the ability to play in a slightly different league. We liked working together; is that enough? Or is it enough to look at what accumulated around the feet of the angel of research, as the funding winds blew her backward into the future, and say: "Well, we published a few papers"? The success of this particular study was not purely in its academic product, not just in the talks we give and the papers we publish.

WHERE WE ARE NOW

By the end of the UARP-funded phase of the UFO study, over 700 young injectors were interviewed, tested, and counseled. Of those who took part in our hepatitis B vaccination follow-up project, about half completed the vaccination series. Both the serological study and the vaccination process have been successfully exported to the Santa

Cruz Needle Exchange, which has become the first needle exchange program in the country to offer this kind of intervention.

In the academic arena, the UFO study staff has presented serological and vaccine data at many national and international conferences (Hahn, Lum, et al., 1999; Hahn, Page-Shafer, Lum, Ochoa, et al., 1999; Lum et al., 1998; Hahn, Lum, et al., 1999; Ochoa, Hahn, Lum, et al., 1999; Ochoa et al., 2001; Page-Shafer et al., 1998; Vadnai et al., 2000). Nine papers have been published or accepted—on HIV serology, HCV serology, HBV vaccine adherence, and overdosing (Davidson et al., 2002, 2003; Evans et al., 2003; Hahn et al., 2002; Lum et al., 2003; Ochoa et al., 2001; Seal et al., 2000; Shafer et al., 2002).

The study has made the transition to the federal level, with a grant from the National Institute on Drug Abuse. The priorities that were defined as a result of our collaborative interaction have become the objectives of this next stage of research, and will remain in our minds for many future endeavors.

REFERENCES

Davidson, P., McLean, R.L., Kral, A.H., Gleghorn, A.A., Edlin, B., and Moss, A.R. (2003). Fatal heroin-related overdose in San Francisco 1997-2000: A case for targeted intervention. *Journal of Urban Health, 80*(2), 261-273.

Davidson, P., Ochoa K.C., Hahn J.A., Evans J.L., and Moss A.R. (2002). Witnessing heroin-related overdoses: The experiences of young injectors in San Francisco. *Addiction, 97*(12), 1511-1516.

Epstein, S. (1996). *Impure Science.* Berkeley: University of California Press.

Evans, J., Hahn, H.A., Page-Shafer, K., Lum, P.J., Stein, E.S., Davidson, P.J., and Moss, A.R. (2003). Gender differences in sexual and injection risk behavior among active young injection drug users in San Francisco (the UFO Study). *Journal of Urban Health, 80*(1), 137-146.

Farmer, P. (1999). *Infections and Inequalities.* Berkeley: University of California Press.

Fernandes, W. and Tandon, R. (1981). *Participatory Research and Evaluation, Experiments in Research As a Process of Liberation.* New Delhi: Indian Social Institute.

Griffiths, P., Gossop, M., Powis, B., and Strang, J. (1993). Reaching hidden populations of drug users by priveleged access interviewers: Methodological and practical issues. *Addiction, 88,* 1617-1626.

Hahn, J., Lum, P., Page-Shafer, K., Ochoa, K., McLean, R., and Moss, A.R. (1999). Access to sterile syringes among young injectors and continued HIV, and hepatitis transmission. Paper presented at the American Public Health Association, 127th Annual Meeting Chicago, Chicago, November.

Hahn, J., Page-Shafer, K., Lum, P.J., Bourgois, P., Stein, E., Evans, J.L., Busch, M.P., Tobler, L.H., Phelps, B., and Moss, A.R. (2002). Hepatitis C virus seroconversion among young injection drug users: Relationships and risks. *Journal of Infectious Diseases, 186*(11), 1558-1564.

Hahn, J., Page-Shafer, K., Lum, P., Ochoa, K., McLean, R., and Moss, A.R. (1999). Viral infections and syringe sharing despite high access to needle exchange. Paper presented at the The Task Force on AIDS and the Universitywide AIDS Research Program Sixteenth Annual Investigators' Meeting and Second Annual Conference on AIDS Research in California, April 16.

Harm Reduction Coalition (1997). *Working Together Toward Individual and Community Health.* New York: Harm Reduction Coalition.

Lum, P., Hahn, J., Page-Shafer, K., Ochoa, K., McLean, R., and Moss, A. (1998). High rates of hepatitis C infection and needle exchange use among young injectors in San Francisco, CA—The UFO Study. Paper presented at the 126th American Public Health Association Annual Meeting, Washington, DC, November.

Lum, P., Ochoa, K., Hahn, J.A., Page-Shafer, K., Evans, J., and Moss, A.R. (2003). Hepatitis B virus immunization among young injection drug users in San Francisco (the UFO Study). *American Journal of Public Health, 93*(6), 919-923.

Lum, P., Ochoa, K., Hahn, J., Page-Shafer, K., McLean, R., and Moss, A. (1999). Low rates of hepatitis B vaccination in young injection drug users in San Francisco. Paper presented at the 127th Annual Meeting of the American Public Health Association, Chicago, November.

Ochoa, K., Hahn, J., Lum, P., Page-Shafer, K., McLean, R., and Moss, A. (1999). Overdose common among young injection drug users. Paper presented at the 127th Annual Meeting of the American Public Health Association, Chicago, November 10.

Ochoa, K., Hahn, J., Seal, K., Lum, P., Page-Shafer, K., McLean, R., and Moss, A. (1999). High HIV risk behavior associated with overdose in young injection drug users. Paper presented at the Sixteenth Annual AIDS Investigators' Meeting and Second Annual Conference on AIDS Research in California, April 16.

Ochoa, K., Hahn, J.A., Seal, K.H., and Moss, A.R. (2001). Overdosing among young injection drug users in San Francisco. *Addict Behavior, 26*(3), 453-460.

Page-Shafer, K., Hahn, J., Ochoa, K., Tulsky, J.P., Sabin, M., Lum, P., McLean, R., and Moss, A. (1998). Prevalence of HIV, HBV, HCV infection in young injectors in San Francisco, CA. Paper presented at the Fifteenth Annual AIDS Investigators' Meeting and First Annual Conference on AIDS Research in California, Los Angeles, California, February.

Seal, K., Ochoa, K.C., Hahn, J.A., Tulsky, J.P., Edlin, B.R., and Moss, A.R. (2000). Risk of hepatitis B infection among young injection drug users in San Francisco: Opportunities for intervention. *West Journal Medicine, 172*(1), 16-20.

Shafer, K., Hahn, J.A., Lum, P.J., Ochoa, K., Graves, A., and Moss, A. (2002). Prevalence and correlates of HIV infection among young injection drug users in San Francisco. *Journal of Acquired Immune Deficiency Syndrome, 31*(4), 422-431.

Vadnai, L., Ochoa, K., Hahn, J.A., Page-Shafer, K., Lum, P.J., Evans, J.L., and Moss, A.R. (2000). Young female injection drug users are younger, have less injection experience than their male counterparts yet have equal rates of HIV, hepatitis B and hepatitis C. Paper presented at the Third Annual Conference on AIDS Research in California and Seventeenth Annual UARP Meeting, San Francisco, February 21.

Chapter 9

Synthesis of Case Studies and Service Providers' Reactions

Benjamin P. Bowser
Lisa M. Krieger

This book describes a model for community-based collaborative research, the community-researcher equal partner collaboration (CREPC) model. Furthermore, it sheds some light on the way social and behavioral sciences are conducted and the way community-based organizations use research. More important, it provides six case histories that test the basic assumptions of the CREPC model. In the first part of this chapter, a meta-analysis of these case histories is presented to provide insights into the efficacy of the CREPC model as a way to facilitate scientifically rigorous research, while maintaining an "equal-partner" collaborative relation with community-based organizations. This includes a discussion of whether CREPC was necessary to make a difference in the quality of the research. By comparing and contrasting the case studies, we outline the principles of successful collaboration and the lessons learned. The six case studies are varied enough in complexity, outcome, and scale to permit study of collaboration as both a research method and a way to enhance service. Did the UARP achieve its goal in funding collaborative research, and were the missions and services of the community-based agencies enhanced by collaboration?

In part two, several community collaborators reflect on their experience with the CREPC model. Rigorous research that is not also useful and enhances services would be inadequate.

PART I: META-ANALYSIS OF CASE STUDIES

Scientifically Rigorous Research?

First, we want to examine the scientific rigor of the six case studies under the CREPC model in terms of their study design, study population, number of collaborators, validity of findings, and range of topics that were and were not investigated. There may be specific topics or research-service situations that collaborative research is particularly useful with and others that it is not. Also important is the issue of scope; does the size and complexity of the project impact the extent of success or failure in collaboration? If not, what are the dimensions that challenge the collaborative framework?

The six case studies provide a broad continuum of design, educational programs, implementation strategies, target populations, and outcomes. The study population in these six studies included young injectors, male-to-female transgender persons, HIV-seropositive prison inmates, HIV high-risk women (injection-drug users, sex workers, and partners of injectors), migrant farmworkers, and street-identified injection-drug users and sex workers. Only two case studies had overlapping study populations, PHREDA and CAL-PEP. PHREDA focused on women and evaluated a health intervention, while CAL-PEP evaluated street outreach services.

The scope of the studies is summarized in Table 9.1.

Design and Populations

CREPC was successfully used for a variety of study designs and study populations. The UFO and transgender studies were epidemiological, and did not use comparison groups. The prison study compared those who received the prerelease training with those who did not. The farmworker study had two experimental and one control group. Those who received all four educational sessions were the first experimental group; the second group consisted of those who received only one session; and the third group was men who received no intervention. In the CAL-PEP study, the outreach clients who received services were compared with those who did not. The number of interviews and persons trained ranged from 123 in the prison study to 696 young adults who were interviewed, tested, and provided services in the UFO study. All of the cases, except the UFO study, had at

TABLE 9.1. Scope of Case Studies

	UFO	Transgender	Prison Inmates	PHREDA	Farmworkers	CAL-PEP
Study design	Epi.**	Epi.**	Panel*	Panel*	Panel*	Panel*
Experimental	None	None	1	None	2	None
Control group	None	None	1	None	1	1
Subject (N =)	696	244	123	327	432	346
Study population	Hi-risk youth	M to F transgender	HIV-positive men	Hi-risk women	Farmworkers	IDUs/sex workers
Pre and posttest	No	Yes	Yes	Yes	Yes	Yes
Bio markers	Yes	Yes	No	No	No	No
Intervention	All	None	Edu	Health	Edu	Outreach
Collaborators	3	4	2	4	2	2
Communities	4	3	1	2	27 camps	2
Services	Yes	No	Yes	Yes	Yes	Yes
Generate data	Yes	Yes	Yes	Yes	Yes	Yes
Significant results	Yes	None	None	Yes	Yes	Yes

*A panel study is a type of longitudinal study in which data are collected from the same sample of persons at several points in time.
**Epi = epidemiology study

least one follow-up interview (posttest) with clients. There were two posttests and a focus group follow-up in the farmworker study.

In the transgender study, there were four collaborators—three community-based agencies (CBOs) and the health department. The PHREDA study included the University of California, San Francisco, Planned Parenthood, and two CBOs. The UFO included two CBOs, the Haight-Ashbury Youth Outreach Team, the Santa Cruz Needle Exchange; and the University of California, San Francisco. The number of communities ranged from one to four, all with drug problems amid high unemployment and high poverty. The San Francisco communities are in early stages of gentrification. In the farmworker study, each of twenty-seven migrant worker camps was counted as a separate community.

Interventions and Significance

In all of the studies, the educational program and/or outreach services with referral constituted the intervention and were evaluated. From the standpoint of research, all of the teams were able to successfully generate data from their interviews and testing. Four of the six studies were able to show statistically significant differences between clients who received services and those who did not. The prison study was a likely victim of low sample size due to the prison administration constraints on intervention. Having statistically significant differences means that the differences between the intervention group and the control group (no intervention) were unlikely to be due to chance. Therefore, the intervention activity is accepted as effective. Where no statistically significant differences existed between the intervention and control groups, the intervention cannot be accepted as having produced an effective outcome.

In PHREDA, there were several statistically significant differences. Those who received services (counseling and physical examinations) were more likely to follow up than those who did not receive services. Farmworkers in the more intense educational program had a more pronounced change in knowledge and, more important, in their behavior. They began using condoms during sex with sex workers, in comparison to workers in the less intense program. In the CAL-PEP study, those who used CAL-PEP outreach services were significantly higher HIV risk takers than those who did not use the services; this was the opposite of what was hypothesized. CAL-PEP outreach services turned out to be very effective in helping street-identified injectors and sex workers significantly reduce and stabilize already high drug use and HIV risks. The PHREDA study of HIV high-risk women had a similar finding of statistically significant numbers of higher risk takers seeking their services. Furthermore, in the CAL-PEP study early adolescent loss through sudden death of close relatives and friends was associated with the highest HIV risk takers. The overall scope of these studies is not outside of the range of most other community studies reported in research journal articles, in which case, any lessons learned here might be transferable to other types of studies with the same scope and range.

Methods

These studies are examples of both qualitative and quantitative research or mixed methods. They are qualitative in that the insights and working knowledge of the service providers and their outreach staffs were identified as if by focus groups and key informants, two of several qualitative methods. They are quantitative in that key insights and ideas are formally tested as research hypotheses and data are generated and analyzed. The CAL-PEP study did this by developing staff-defined research hypotheses. Staff insights were also essential in the organization and successful conduct of the farmworker, prison, transgender, and UFO studies. None of the studies did formal ethnography prior to colleting data.

In effect, the prior experiences of program staff were used as observational data to derive insight about their clients and to suggest the best way to organize a more structurally grounded research experience. The whole point of any qualitative research is to generate insights about the study population. In mixed methodologies, the insights are used to develop the quantitative phase of the research. Here the quantitative design is grounded in the reality of the people one wished to recruit and interview, and there is the potential to supplement the former theory and questions with new questions and theory based on the qualitative insights. But the role of qualitative research does not stop here. In mixed designs, there are potential points during the quantitative phase of the research when additional insights and "feedback" from staff and subject-clients can be incorporated into the interviews and then later in data analysis.

Ongoing concerns and insights from the transgender interviewers pointed out that the interviews were not emotionally neutral events. Clients often needed counseling afterward. This point certainly confirmed the efficiency of the questions, alerted the principal investigators of a potential follow-up issue, and suggested that they had other issues yet to formally explore. As the staff in the UFO study identified new issues outside of the initial scope of the study, the new issues were incorporated into the study making it more humane and useful to clients not only as research, but also as a service improvement.

Furthermore, all of the teams generated quantitative data to evaluate their intervention and service, and to gain new insight and ideas for further exploration. The UFO project was the only one that did not study an intervention. The process of moving from qualitative to quantitative methods and back again addresses two problems in research methods. First, qualitative research focused on keeping the researcher grounded in the reality, issues, and concerns of those being studied. For research to be relevant, potentially useful, and meaningful, it must be "grounded." That is, the hypotheses, variables, and analyses must be about the real things of real people, not just the researchers' theoretical construct of reality and people. The mixed method approach in these studies does this.

In quantitative research the problem arises of successive studies to improve and advance research hypotheses and their underlying theory. Rarely in the social and behavioral sciences is any subject studied repeatedly under the very same study conditions. Even when the same people are reinterviewed two or more times, their experiences between times and the conditions they respond under differ from interview to interview. Mixed methods research allows investigators to do research as a dynamic event in which new factors can be incorporated in the same study and across studies. Each study continues to be unique but each study is able to better capture the factors that make their clients and results unique for the moment and circumstance. In doing so, the research enterprise is advanced.

What Differences Does CREPC Make in Research Quality?

The most important research issue regarding the scope of these case studies is the extent to which they were able to be equal partner collaborative projects. As pointed out in both Chapters 1 and 2, the UARP collaborative research projects were not the first collaborative projects. Research-CBO collaborations are increasingly popular, and are largely driven by funding agencies' increasing demand for accountability through evaluation of social service agencies. Collaborations are also driven by the critical need for effective prevention of a host of communicable diseases in hard-to-access groups. What is distinct about the UARP projects is that they were very consciously designed to be *equal partner collaborations* between community-based social service agencies and researchers (CREPC).

Research collaborations have traditionally been characterized by a "top-down" and "research expertise" approach. Governmental agencies frequently act as the research authority and use CBOs as field sites for their agenda in a top-down approach. If field sites have the ability to supplement the government-sponsored research with their own studies, they can do so. But most often the agency gives the basic research model to the CBO with little opportunity to provide feedback that would then be used as a necessary part of the partnership to enhance and better ground the research protocol.

Other research collaborations have been characterized by the "division of labor" or "research expertise" approach. This approach is based upon prior work in technical transfer and action research (Binson et al., 1997; Gómez and Goldstein, 1995). Researchers with this background frame their role as providing research expertise to conduct evaluations of CBO services and programs. Although some of these partnerships may evolve into true collaborations, the "research expertise" approach does not formally assume that the community partner will be brought into the research planning, development of hypotheses, and conduct of the research. This is an improvement over the top-down model.

In contrast to the top-down and the expertise models, CREPC collaborations very consciously make the research and community partner equal in contribution and dependent upon one another to improve the quality of the research as well as the utility of the final outcome for the agencies; prior community-based research that used collaboration has shown the necessity of such well-articulated equal partnerships (Israel et al., 1998). So, to what extent were the UARP case studies equal partner collaborations?

All of the case studies in this collection satisfied the basic criteria outlined in Chapter 1. One criterion in particular needs to be discussed. To ensure the selection of successful collaborations, the UARP peer review process included evaluation criteria based on the quality of the proposed collaboration and the collaborators' prior experience working in collaboration. All six teams had prior working experiences as collaborators. This was a very important factor that influenced data and project outcomes. In the CAL-PEP, farmworker, PHREDA, prison, and UFO studies, the equal partners had prior histories of collaboration; in some cases, the collaborators had years of prior experience with one another. The only project in which no long-term prior experience occurred between partners was the transgender study. Furthermore, the six cases were not the only community-researcher collaborations for either partner in most of the studies. In this sense, the UARP selection criteria stacked the deck with highly selective projects.

Challenges to Collaboration

Regardless of the partners' backgrounds, the initial selection criteria were challenged in the actual conduct of each project. Each project was more or less challenged to maintain its balance between partners. In which case, maintaining equal partner collaboration was a moving target and required a great deal of flexibility and problem solving on the part of collaborators. The following is an illustration of the extent to which the case studies achieved equal partnerships in their actual conduct.

UFO

The UFO study was the most radical in its efforts to maintain balance between partners. All staff considered themselves equal partners, and came closest of all of the studies to being staff and client driven. The equal partner collaboration was not simply between the researcher and CBO director; all of the staff felt that they had an equal say. This is largely a reflection of the CBO's prior operating culture as a flat hierarchy. This posed an extreme challenge to the research partner who had to convince everyone in the project of the efficiency of all the research requirements.

"Equal partner" staff extended the partnership envelope to include actively drug-using clients as well. Actively using clients became part of the outreach and interviewer teams. Alternatively, a flat hierarchy has advantages. Once everyone has bought in, it engenders a high level of commitment from everyone involved. Not many projects could lay off their staff and have them show up the next morning ready to work because of dedication to the project and their clients. Also, the CBO put its access to young injectors and its reputation on the line to enforce eligibility requirements for study participation. The CBO was willing to risk failing in its central mission in order to support the project. Here again, the commitment to the research was extraordinary.

Transgender

In the transgender study the three CBOs facilitated the research as an extension of their outreach activities. But only one CBO was a coordinating partner. This is an interesting case of one CBO working to motivate and involve two others across the race and community spectrum. There were tensions between them. But it appears that open lines of communications were helpful through periodic and open meetings for feedback from all of the CBO staff. An important factor in the success of this project to accommodate its unequal community partners was that the interviewers, although part of the research team, were based in the three CBO communities. They worked with all three CBO outreach teams and, in doing so, provided continuity and unity in the field. It was also helpful that the interview team was proactive and gave suggestions about improving the conduct of the study. In effect, all of the community partners were not equal partners in the organization of the project, but they had to be involved in the successful conduct of each project.

CAL-PEP

As in the transgender study, the CAL-PEP interviewers were specifically hired and worked with the regular CAL-PEP outreach teams.

Periodic joint-partner meetings were held to identify problems and to work on consensus solutions. The CAL-PEP collaboration was less complex than the transgender study in that there was only one CBO. Clients were not equal partners, but their concerns were represented by CAL-PEP staff, a number of whom were former clients.

Farmworker Study

The farmworker study paralleled both the transgender and CAL-PEP studies with two differences. In the farmworkers' study, the outreach workers also served as interviewers and trainers, and like CAL-PEP, there was only one CBO collaborator. The second difference is that the project was challenged by farm owners who were concerned that the health outreach staff persons were also union organizers. It is remarkable that the study was completed as designed under the circumstance.

Prison Study

The prison study was a model collaboration between a CBO and a research partner, both of whom had worked together before. The challenge to their project came from the prison administration. The CBO was extraordinary in the first place for being able to negotiate access to prisoners, but what the CBO was not able to control were prison administrative decisions that repeatedly compromised access to the prisoners. The prison study collaborative team had to periodically redesign their project around prison directives. Each time, their project design was compromised.

PHREDA

The third phase of the PHREDA project was to get HIV high-risk women into health treatment. The equal partner collaboration was between a university partner and Planned Parenthood served as the community partner. But two CBOs, which were not equal partners, were the field sites and service partners. PHREDA was challenged when Planned Parenthood reorganized and got new leadership. In the meantime, they did not work closely enough with one of the field-site community partners. That partner dropped out of the project because their concerns and issues were not addressed. Here again, a project design was compromised and had to be scaled back.

The lesson is that whenever parties are not engaged at some important level in the project, potential exists for surprise and disruption that may lead to a compromise of the research design. In theory, it is in the best interest of complex community-based research to involve as many parties with disruptive potentials as possible in the project.

Was CREPC Sufficient?

All of UARP's central criteria for collaborative research were met despite challenges to the process in several studies. All of the partners had a common goal of slowing, if not preventing the spread of HIV/AIDS. Each partner understood that they needed each other to successfully slow down or prevent the spread of HIV. The researchers and CBO directors were equal partners. All of the partners were equally involved initially in planning their projects. Each team had a mutual understanding of the end products.

The next requirement was absolutely essential and needs to be highlighted. Mutual trust was imperative, along with regular meetings to address problems, and openness and flexibility in problem solving. All of the projects were challenged on this point and had repeated issues to resolve. In the UFO study all of the initial and ongoing staff concerns regarding research had to be addressed, and based upon their experience interviewing clients, UFO moved to incorporate HCV, HBV, and overdose prevention into their initial HIV investigation. Problem solving in the transgender study led to interviewers being trained in outreach safety procedures, and to one interviewer challenging the nature of one of the agency's transgender services. In the prison study, the prison periodically moved prisoners, and did security lockdowns requiring the team to adapt their research and program procedures. This required a great deal of flexibility and skill to keep the project alive as research. One of the community collaborators dropped out of PHREDA precisely because it felt that Planned Parenthood, being reorganized and with new leadership, was unresponsive to its concerns. The farmworker study had to exercise great diplomacy and flexibility over the indefiniteness of access to work camps. Depending on the sensitivities and concerns of the owners and overseers, their educational sites were periodically opened or closed to the research team for essential follow-ups. In the CAL-PEP study tensions between the outreach and interview teams had to be resolved as well as damage control from one interviewer who did fraudulent initial interviews.

Finally, there is an area in which several projects were most successful. Community collaborators contributed to the research questions and had their insights tested in addition to having their program evaluated and client epidemiology measured. The UFO study extended the scope of its research to include HCV and HBV testing and overdose prevention based upon the community partners' concerns. In the CAL-PEP study, the community partner and outreach staff helped define half of the etiology research questions and hypotheses. CAL-PEP staff also made certain that clients would recognize the research questions about program components by their street names. In the farmworker study, cultural competency was very effectively addressed through the use of *fotonovela*, and *radionovela*, as well as Spanish-speaking interviewers and outreach staff. This study could not have been possible without culturally competent staff and research instruments that took into consideration the client literacy levels. The transgender study questions required the involvement of transgender people. People outside of this community are simply not knowledgeable enough of both the physical and social-emotional issues involved in male-to-female transitions.

Other Factors

The UARP provided excellent guidelines to produce projects that would innovate collaboration and have potential to produce quality data and improve service program outcomes. But as discussed earlier, the initial program guidelines may not have been sufficient to produce the end result. Once these projects were underway, other unanticipated factors influenced outcomes. We learned enough about the processes in most of these projects to isolate some other unanticipated factors.

Continuous Training

Part of the success of the CAL-PEP and farmworker studies was continuous staff training. In both projects, the regular staff meetings were used to train staff about research as well as to problem solve and troubleshoot. In the CAL-PEP study this included two teams—the outreach recruiters and the interviewers. In the farmworker study, the AIDS service organization outreach team members were also the intervention trainers and interviewers. In retrospect, neither research principal investigator set out with a curriculum. Training occurred as a part of the definition of their role in the project, a definition that was defined and permitted by their service organization coprincipal investigator. In both cases, the service organization staff became much more sophisticated about research by the end of the UARP project. The AIDS service coprincipal investigator in the farmworker study returned to school for an advanced degree, and the CAL-PEP staff went on to write research proposals and to receive funding for several subsequent grants with evaluation requirements. The more radical UFO project has gone on to be funded as a NIDA RO1, the most competitive of NIDA research funding. Despite initial reservations about research, staff on the UFO project became quite knowledgeable about research.

Visibility with Staff

The extent to which the research and CBO partners were directly involved in the project also impacted research outcomes. The research and CBO partners set the stage for staff to execute the projects. A crucial level of visibility was essential for team morale and provided another level of accessibility for problem identification and solution, and training. Staff was not left alone for very long without feedback and the opportunity to provide feedback. In the early stages of each project, close supervision was essential. Virtually every problem in the field across all of these projects could be traced to periods when either the research or CBO partners were not visible such as in the CAL-PEP study when an interviewer attempted to complete questionnaires himself, and in PHREDA when a site withdrew from the study because its issues were not addressed. Also, the less experienced the staff in conducting interviews, the more supervision they needed.

The inner conduct of the research is one thing, but the experiences and impressions of the service collaborators could be quite different. In this sense, a review of the conduct of these projects would be incomplete without assessments.

PART II: ASSESSING CREPC

CREPC Intervention Assessments

The complexities of people's lives are often lost in current approaches to research. As a result, research has not sufficiently helped high-risk communities—and communities have not contributed to research. By blending science and sociology, merging the rigor of survey techniques with the subtleties of human insight, AIDS prevention efforts can be improved by becoming better targeted.

Until recently, science and community collaborations have been rare. Moreover, the community and scientific researchers come from two distinct cultures. Historically, people in the community have believed that researchers lack insight into their lives. They may resist volunteering in studies due to their involvement in illegal activities involving sex and drugs. Even if community groups sought to conduct research or were required to monitor their work by funding agencies, they often lacked the time, money, and staff to do so.

However, at the same time, community-based activists recognize the value that researchers bring to their programs. Without scientific expertise, there is no way to prove that their programs are making a difference. Even if community programs are proven effective in one setting, research findings may help them demonstrate that they are equally effective in another. Research offers them a tool and methodology to measure their services and prove that they are meeting a community's changing needs. It might also show where they could improve and better focus their attention. Our community collaborators testify to this fact:

"A collaboration can improve both the research and community side of the work," states Cathy J. Reback, director of the Prevention Division of Van Ness Recovery House in West Hollywood (Chapter 6). "From the community perspective, interventions and instruments can be improved when the community partners realize how their services can turn into data and be used for the greater good. From the research perspective, I believe that research can only improve by spending time in the community and actually learning about the population."

For such collaborations to work, the goals of both researchers and communities must be equally served. The goal of the researcher is to improve the quality of the science, yielding findings that will be truly useful for the prevention of HIV or other social problems. The goal of the community is to improve services, work more effectively with clients, and demonstrate the value of their work. "Before collaboration is launched," notes Reback, "the researcher must first ask, 'What questions do we want answered?' . . . And community partners must ask, 'What roles can a researcher play in my agency?'"

Despite their substantial benefits, collaborations pose significant challenges. Collaborations are expensive and time-consuming, often straining already limited resources. Collaborations run counter to the procedures and identities of both types of organizations. Moreover, their distinct cultures can create a huge gulf between groups who need each other's expertise and access but find themselves in separate philosophical and political camps.

Because disenfranchised communities have traditionally lacked access to political power or health care, they may be suspicious of research projects. Moreover, their behaviors and sexual identities can be difficult to measure using traditional tools. The methodologically rigorous approach required for research can interfere with provision of important services. Fernando Sanudo of the Vista Community Clinic's Health Promotion Program, who worked in migrant farmworker communities (Chapter 4), states:

> We can certainly learn from each other's area of expertise but trust must be developed first. Traditionally, there has not been a lot of trust between these two fields. What we learned in the transgender study was that the trust started with learning about each other's culture, such as their dress and language.

Powerful research institutes, whose primary purpose is to generate knowledge, are positioned outside the real life of HIV risk takers and the people who work directly with them on prevention. In order for researchers' work to withstand the scrutiny of peers, they seek rigorous application of the scientific method. Concerns about the quality of their research lead them to want to maintain control over research environments. This tendency conflicts directly with the need for prevention programs and with the dynamics of community groups where autonomy is highly valued. According to Sanudo,

Understanding these challenges, academic researchers need to adapt the overall research protocol to better meet the needs of the research participants and community health workers. The willingness of researchers to change their research designs [will] better serve the population. . . . The needs of the population and community health workers need to be given more priority than a research framework as designed on paper.

The collaboration between an AIDS service organization and an academic institution creates "systems change" between partners. For instance, academic researchers are forced to understand the realities of outreach and other challenges faced by community workers when collecting data for the purposes of research. . . . Understanding these challenges, academic researchers need to adapt the overall research protocol to better meet the needs of the research participants and community health workers.

Community-based input can be difficult to sustain due to changes in staff, office relocation, and other turbulence. In addition, external factors can disrupt research. Problems experienced by researchers, as documented in this book, range from farm owners physically threatening the lives of outreach workers to sudden prison inmate relocations.

Because race and/or class may also separate community activists and researchers, subtle tensions may exist in their relationship. A quiet struggle over issues of power and authority, exacerbated by historic economic or racial inequality may underlie even the best collaboration.

Collaborations work best when, despite their challenges, scientists and community activists work as equal partners in an investigation, both are involved in defining and conducting research.

To make the relationship work, both sides need to identify each other's goals and expectations. They must educate themselves about each other's needs and procedures. The best partnerships are created when researchers and activists work together on a project's survey design, and develop and implement the protocol. Partners must decide, jointly, how to define research questions, create a methodology, and build a shared understanding of how research findings will be used. Some special training of staff may prove necessary. Community members who teach may have to become more assertive. They must understand the goals of research and resist emotional involvement with the community they are studying. Fernando Sanudo states:

> To make a collaboration succeed, the AIDS service organization (ASO) must be involved in the entire project—from planning to evaluation. . . . They must also have an opportunity to learn how to conduct evaluations, so they grasp the terminology and research design. With their trust, HIV prevention services are greatly improved.
>
> In an atmosphere of mutual trust and respect, it is important to acknowledge the two different agendas: methodological rigor versus flexibility. A common language may be necessary, avoiding both the jargon of researchers and the vernacular of the community. And each side must be sensitive to stresses within both organizations. . . . Researchers need to understand a relationship between the community health workers and target populations, so not to alienate or jeopardize their relationship.

Underlying each effort should be a philosophical shift away from "business as usual." Both sides must share the strong belief that the quality of social science theory is vastly improved when it is built upon the study of practical problems from the community's perspective. Research becomes a tool for broadening the understanding of social problems.

With the help of the community, scientists can gain insights into clients, exploring more deeply their work and family backgrounds. Assistance by scientists aids community groups in gaining empowerment and increasing organizational competence and effectiveness. Collaborations help scientists develop innovative, reliable, and valid data collection techniques. They gain experience in serving a high-risk population. Despite the technical and logistical challenges of conducing collaborative projects, partnerships offer important insights into improved research strategies. Collaborations open doors to new research questions, and offer future opportunities that would go unrecognized if scientists stayed in their offices.

Through collaboration, researchers learn how to better tailor an intervention—rather than imposing an intervention and then demanding that the population accept it. This can improve outreach and the likelihood that services will meet clients' needs.

The community gains something from collaboration as well. With the expertise and expanded support of researchers, the community may be able to expand its programs to additional sites, introducing new people to programs. They gain training in how to conduct a research study. For future funding, they can offer higher quality proposals. Their programs can be more easily marketed due to widespread community support.

"For an AIDS service organization, collaboration forces a change in the way an intervention is implemented," states Sanudo. Historically, limited funding has forced ASOs to develop interventions that are quick and easy. "Not enough time has been devoted to collecting data to determine whether or not an intervention actually influences behavior," he notes. Too often, ASOs have relied on verbal feedback and anecdotal information from the people they serve.

Furthermore, collaboration also forces community health workers to discuss the importance of evaluating the effectiveness of their programs. As a result, they are able to modify or adapt the intervention, so as to decrease the risky behaviors of those they are trying to help. Not only is there a change in the type of intervention—but evaluations are incorporated into subsequent programs.

A synergy can take place, enhancing performance and increasing opportunities due to joint trainings, coordination of activities, and shared space, materials, and staff. Access to funding is improved for both the community-based partners and researchers; they are able to attain support not otherwise available.

For Reback and her staff, the long-term impact of the collaboration on transgender health has been felt in two areas. First, the study provided the community with data on transgender health issues such as sociodemographics, HIV seroprevalence, STD incidence, violence, drug use, and sexual risks that could be used by the community in grant development, program design, working with law officials, and in future conferences. Second, the study bonded the transgender community, leading to the creation of a transgender consortium as well as several transgender community events. Reback states,

> In our situation the project could not have taken off without a partnership. In other situations, where a project can exist independent from a collaboration, I feel a partnership can serve to make a study or an intervention more responsive to both sides.

The multiplicity of approaches to solving social and health problems, as described by this book, proves that no single prevention measure reduces risk. Together, they offer a powerful advantage in the war against disease or addiction.

The projects portrayed here helped change behavior, reduced HIV risk, and slowed the spread of the HIV virus. These collaborations may have prevented the spread of AIDS to many lives. In addition, the accumulation of data could play an important role in improving the quality of future HIV prevention services.

However, its lessons are not confined to AIDS. This approach, replicated elsewhere, can be applied to the design of programs that tackle ill health, substandard housing, dirty water, substance abuse, mental disorders, and other social and public health problems.

Collaboration creates a deeper understanding of people at risk. It keeps research responsive to the needs of the community and it creates a long-standing relationship to build on in the future.

Complex challenges require collective, not isolated, action.

REFERENCES

Binson, D., Harper, G., Grinstead, O., and Haynes-Sanstad, K. (1997). The center for AIDS prevention studies' collaboration program: An alliance of AIDS scientists and community-based organizations. In A.F.P. Nyden, M. Shibley, and D. Borrows (Eds.), *Building Community: Social Science in Action* (pp. 177-189). Thousand Oaks, CA: Pine Forge Press.

Gómez, C. and Goldstein, E. (1995). The HIV prevention evaluation initiative: A model for collaborative evaluation. In D.M. Fetterman, S.J. Kaftarian, and A. Wandersman (Eds.), *Empowerment and Evaluation: Knowledge and Tools for Self-Assessment and Accountability* (pp. 100-122). Thousand Oaks, CA: Sage Publications.

Israel, B., Schulz, A.J., Parker, E.A., and Becker, A. (1998). Review of community-based research: Assessing partnership approaches to improve public health. *Annual Review of Public Health, 19,* 173-202.

Chapter 10

Conclusion

Benjamin P. Bowser
Shiraz I. Mishra
Cathy J. Reback
George F. Lemp

THE CHALLENGE

HIV/AIDS kills by spreading silently, exploiting our most basic human vulnerabilities: sex practices, secrets about sexuality, addictions to drugs, poor self-image, and denial. The emotions aroused by sexuality can play havoc with reason. Many people think that HIV infection is a disease affecting only drug addicts, gay men, and African Americans. They believe that it is unlikely that someone who is not a drug injector and not gay can acquire HIV. Still others think that if their sexual partner does not look "sick," HIV cannot be passed on to them.

The HIV virus does not confine itself to those already impacted by it. It is true that the majority of those infected are men who have sex with men, African Americans, the poor, and drug injectors. But what is not understood is that these are not populations isolated from general society; HIV high-risk behaviors overlap race and class boundaries. As with other diseases, Americans with the least access to clean and safe environments, health care, and prevention knowledge are infected first. Whatever the disease, people on the margins of society are more vulnerable and suffer the greatest harm. African Americans, men who have sex with men, drug injectors, and the poor are more connected to all of society than most imagine. Groups of people may discriminate against one another and believe that their race, class, sexual preference, and community keep them separate, but the HIV virus honors no such boundaries. If HIV/AIDS risks continue to be ignored among the most vulnerable, HIV will slowly and silently continue to spread to other populations within society, maintaining the epidemic for future generations.

AIDS is tragic not because it is inevitable and cannot be stopped. The spreading AIDS pandemic is tragic precisely because it is 100 percent preventable. The millions of deaths, related losses, and suffering are unnecessary. Furthermore, although we are able to keep those infected with HIV alive with new wonder drugs—protease inhibitors and others—access to these therapies and the proper management of them is limited to a fraction of those infected worldwide.

Since AIDS kills and will not be confined only to the most vulnerable populations, effective action is necessary to prevent it. People need to be educated, reeducated, and educated again. Social norms that allow sexual exploitation and encourage drug use and abuse must be changed. Also, factors which compel people to inject drugs and share needles must be addressed. The clock is running; "business as usual" will not work. Prevention is urgent and calls for the best that we have—science, insight, prayers, art for inspiration, and luck. If our prevention tools are insufficient, then we must invent more effective ones. Whole generations are at stake. They will continue to suffer if we maintain "business as usual."

If we remain unconvinced that HIV/AIDS is a major threat, other related disease pandemics will manifest in the not-too-distant future (Horowitz, 1997; Morse, 1993). These new diseases will be equally as baffling as AIDS and will also challenge our intellect, science, preventive efforts, and ultimately our humanity toward one another. So we must "get it right" with AIDS, because similar preventive efforts may be essential for stemming the course of future diseases and pandemics.

The prevention research projects described in this book were inspired by this sense of urgency, a recognition that this work had to be done. The usual research methods and social service constraints could no longer stand in the way. We had to create high-quality science and prevention services simultaneously; one could not proceed without the other. The promise of science is its ability to improve the effectiveness of social services. Thus, we had to solve an organizational problem to ultimately improve outcomes for people at high risk for HIV infection.

No one got wealthy, more comfortable, or famous doing this work. Motivated by necessity, we learned a new way to do science and social services and have advanced a human technology with applications well beyond AIDS prevention. *Equal partner collaborative research* has enormous implications for improving the outcomes of a host of other social problems in the United States and the rest of the world—housing, homelessness, ethnic relations, and crime, just to name a few. Enormous implications exist for improving commercial research and marketing. No magic is involved here, just the need to change researchers' attitudes toward the people under study and engage them as equal partners. If successful, the science improves, the services improve, and people's lives are improved. If the most vulnerable people can prevent AIDS in their own lives and the lives of those close to them, then together we can do almost anything.

In this final chapter, we review why innovation is necessary in how we conduct research and provide social services and why equal partner collaboration is one such innovation. Then we discuss how to proceed in the future. Equal partner collaboration is not the end all. We need more innovations and more imaginative work to improve the effectiveness of science and social services collaborations.

BUSINESS AS USUAL

It is hard to imagine a nation of over 270 million people living in an economy dedicated to individual advancement and profit that adequately cares for the health and human needs of its most vulnerable citizens. Even in a global capitalist system, some form of social services is needed. Traditionally, the government protects those in need and provides them with necessary services. However, with the collapse of the Soviet Union and the socialist alternative economy and social system, the United States is slowly dismantling its welfare system because there is no alternative model that shows better results. Welfare in the new world order is too expensive and ineffective. This includes the public medical system.

Even if the medical system that provides for the poor remained intact, it is not sufficient to prevent the continued spread of AIDS. The most vulnerable people have multiple problems. They need safe housing, income to buy food and clothing, education and job training, child care services, legal assistance, and psychological counseling. AIDS outreach workers know that the prevention message goes nowhere as long as their clients' more basic and immediate needs are unmet. It is difficult to care about a disease that causes death in ten years if you currently suffer from inadequate shelter, food, income, and self-worth. People at highest risk of HIV infection do whatever they have to do to survive now and worry about long-term consequences of their risks later.

AIDS outreach workers work in a "catch-22 area." To be effective, they must help address their clients' basic human needs. Yet AIDS outreach workers are trained and funded to only deal with AIDS prevention. The "business as usual" approach taken by CBOs has a basic organizational flaw: their funding is organized by distinct categories of need. Although convenient to the U.S. Congress, this translates into fragmented services to people in need. So if one needs help, it is necessary to apply for housing at one site, get food stamps someplace else, travel across town to get to a health clinic, receive drug treatment at another site, then get job training in yet another location. It is a full-time job to travel from office to office and stand in long lines in each location. In addition, people seeking help must keep up with applications and requirements that are often contradictory; all of this must be done between 9 a.m. and 5 p.m., despite the fact that most poor have to work during these hours. They lose income, perhaps even lose their jobs, by taking time off. If any service is to be effective, it must be available where and when people need it. Services should also be comprehensive.

Coinciding with this dismantling of marginal public health services, is an AIDS epidemic. These trends are on a collision course—and if we have "business as usual," AIDS will win. Government involvement cannot be circumvented, either through direct services or indirectly by funding private nonprofits. HIV prevention must be part of a comprehensive package of human services. From whatever perspective, there are no profits in AIDS prevention outside of government involvement and subsidy.

Needless to say, HIV prevention funding is not extensive enough to meet the growing need—and the gap is widening. The deficiency is most obvious in the organizations that support outreach. This organizational front line consists primarily of underfunded, understaffed, one-service community-based organizations—AIDS service organizations (ASOs). Their equivalent organization within city public health departments is the equally underfunded and understaffed "AIDS Division." Most organizations that offer drug treatment, affordable housing, mental health services, legal counsel, job training, adult literacy, and other services are similarly stretched. It is rare for an ASO to be large enough to provide multiple services. So the AIDS front line is no different from the front line for all other social services in the United States—it is business as usual. At some point, this public policy-driven impasse must be addressed.

Even if sufficient funding is available, an additional problem exists. The effectiveness of HIV/AIDS prevention programs is generally unknown. We cannot expect prevention to work if the effectiveness of the frontline efforts is unmeasured. The problem warrants the highest level of effectiveness and a new understanding of organizations. All programmatic activities must be continuously evaluated—not for the sake of researchers' careers, but because the organization needs it. This evaluation must be continuous and used to improve program activity.

To achieve this level of self-examination and ongoing change, several barriers must be broken. The first barrier is the well-founded suspicion of CBOs (and ASOs) about science and scientists. Many community practitioners believe that researchers lack knowledge and insight about their lives, and still worse, do not care about anything other than their next publication. They believe that science is inflexible, overly complex, impossible to understand, requires advanced degrees, and is detached from the community. They believe, in effect, that research is irrelevant to serving real people. The second barrier is the attitude of many scientists toward their work and community. They believe that only scientists can do research and must fully control their projects. In this view people are subjects or "organisms," and communities are only field sites. All ideas and influences that are not part of their research protocol create bias and result in "noise" in the data.

Where such extreme attitudes exist, the advancement of knowledge about people, their motives, and their behaviors suffers. Also, social service programs operate largely in the dark with regard to their effectiveness due to lack of ongoing evaluation. They must rely upon episodic cases and faith that their work makes a difference.

Again, this is business as usual and is totally inadequate to stop the AIDS epidemic.

Obviously the community needs to become more central to research efforts. Service agencies must participate in research not simply to create new theory but to create solutions to social problems. This requires community people to become full partners and collaborators in defining research hypotheses, project design, and in executing the work and interpreting the results. Researchers need to use their knowledge to rigorously and sensitively evaluate program efforts. They must persist during the process of revision and improvement that results from their evaluations, and then repeat the cycle again. This improves both science and practice. The projects described in this book provide illustrations of such work and improvements.

NEW BUSINESS:
GROUNDED RESEARCH AND SERVICES

Any efforts to stop the AIDS epidemic among vulnerable populations before it reaches the general society will require reorganizing the administration of social services and rethinking how organizational evaluations are done. Social services in the United States are ineffective because they are not organized to assist those in need; they are not "grounded." The U.S. Congress is far removed from service providers and those in need in the flatlands of Oakland, the Haight-Ashbury neighborhood of San Francisco, Harlem in New York, the South Side of Chicago, and the migrant worker fields of Southern California. By the time money and regulations work their way down to the states, cities, and counties, then to the funding administrations, and finally to the community-based agencies, it is a miracle that anyone is helped.

The reorganization of social services will require rebuilding the provision of services from the level of the client *up,* not from Congress *down.* Fragmentation of needs must be reduced. Ideally, a person would have all of his or her needs assessed and addressed at one time. Services should be made available where and when clients can receive them. This might mean, for instance, using mobile vans with comprehensive caseworkers who can do full assessments and complete applications on the streets after midnight. Similarly, medical and prevention services could be made available by mobile vans after hours in the neighborhoods of high-risk people, such as migrant worker camps and streets frequented by sex traders, homeless youth, and transgender people. If it is possible to effectively use marketing to target consumers of soap, cars, food, and other products, it can be done with comprehensive human services. As in the most effective sales and services, the client may not always be "right," but the client certainly must come first, and before the convenience of the vendor or government bureaucracy.

Science needs a similar grounding. As part of the larger struggle to combat the AIDS epidemic, scientists must become more engaged in evaluating HIV prevention services. As outlined in Chapter 1, there is a long history in the social and behavioral sciences of debate and slow progress regarding the extent to which scientists engage in society. Traditionalists hold that the pursuit of scientific knowledge about human behavior and society comes first—and must be separate from politics or ideologies. According to this perspective, the scientist must fully control research in order for free inquiry to take place. Traditionalists follow the model of the bench sciences in fields such as physics and chemistry, where investigators have full control over the chemicals, materials, forces, and conditions of research. Their dream is to do the same in human society.

Since people and society are more than chemicals, materials, and forces, nontraditional scientists who see the limits of "pure" science wish to devise ways to engage people in their full complexity and spirit. Whatever makes humans behave in certain ways will not be understood by dissection. To understand and perhaps change human behavior, people must be engaged as participants in their own study. The job of the scientists with regard to HIV high risk, for example, is to guide high-risk takers through defining, describing, testing, and analyzing their own behaviors and motives. This is not easy. It requires understanding the principles of science as well as any traditionalist, but also being capable of engaging people fully; the science and social engagement must work simultaneously. This embeds scientific findings in the reality of the people and social settings it wishes to understand. Then we create the possibility of learning how to convince people to change their behavior, even a behavior as deeply personal as sex or drug use. "Equal partner collaboration" is a step toward such an application of science.

EQUAL PARTNER COLLABORATION

The principles of equal partner collaboration were summarized in Chapter 1.

The application of these principles runs counter to the cultures and identities of both research and social service organizations. It consumes more time and requires constant training and monitoring of new interviewers and outreach workers. It is a difficult process to sustain and easy to disrupt both from within and without. Equal partner collaboration can potentially transcend or accommodate differences in community, race, and social class.

The researchers and community service participants whose work was reviewed in this book will testify that collaboration is well worth the cost. The work of the service organizations was evaluated as needed. But in addition, hypotheses about clients were tested and new insights were generated—accomplishments which could not have been achieved by conducting "business as usual." The researchers accumulated better data and gained important insights about hard-to-access groups due to the intimate involvement of the service agency; for their part, community agencies were able to improve services.

Equal partner collaborative research expands the range of applications for social and behavioral research, and provides some assurance that the results will be useful. It also gives community service organizations the assurance that any research done on their clients and involving their services will seek and respect the agencies' and clients' realities. The ultimate result is information about an agency's clients, and its effectiveness, that can be understood and used. This is particularly important due to the vast difference between the disenfranchised communities of HIV risk takers and powerful research institutions.

Powerful outcomes in addition to improved services and research can also be realized. The shift in how things are done for both the service agency and researcher is applicable beyond the immediate project. At a time of increasing frustration and skepticism about the limits of public policy, it is possible to develop a new belief in the relevance of the social sciences. Theories are vastly improved when they are based upon the study of problems from a community organization's perspective. In addition, equal partner collaborations become a tool for broadening our understanding of social problems, potentially offering new solutions. Researchers can gain improved insights about hard-to-reach high-risk clients and can more thoroughly test existing and past ideas. Community organizations are empowered in their work by increasing the skill, competency, and effectiveness of staff.

Additional benefits can also be achieved. The staff learns to do interviews and to better understand research. Funding proposals are of higher quality. There is increased justification for external funding and support. New services can be introduced; existing services can be refined. The organization stays current and learns to tailor interventions to its clients' needs, rather than impose an intervention and demand that clients accept it. There is less risk of losing touch with a community's service population or of imposing an intervention that no longer works or is presented in a way that offends clients. Finally, as in the case of the University of California University-wide AIDS Research Program collaborative research initiative, new funding is accessed that neither the researcher nor the community can obtain alone.

Collaboration offers researchers innovative directions for their research, participation in a direct application of science, and new insights about research strategies. The ability to collect reliable data on hidden and hard-to-reach populations is a major achievement in itself. Moreover, participants are motivated to give accurate responses when the project is based upon a long-term relationship between a community partner and client population. That is not all. The research team gains cultural competence through its work with participants and becomes more highly motivated.

FINAL WORD: THIS IS ONLY A BEGINNING

What we have defined and demonstrated in this book is only a beginning. Potential benefits (and drawbacks) may be found to other types of collaborations between parties who act as equal partners and do research. For example, the potential exists to create equal partner collaborations between social service agencies that offer different categorical services. What would happen, for instance, if HIV/AIDS prevention workers teamed up with those who offer medical, housing, or mental health services? What if researchers also joined in this new collaboration between categorical agencies—and could measure the comparative effectiveness of the combined services, in contrast to single and separate services?

The equal partner collaboration demonstrated in this book was incomplete. It was hard for researchers and community service people to work in collaboration. How much harder would it be, and what would be the benefits of including clients as equal partners in research and evaluation? Service agencies are islands of stability in seemingly chaotic worlds of sex traders, injection-drug users, migrant workers, women who inject drugs, and transgender people. But would we gain even greater insights and more useful perspectives on the social problems of these populations by training their members to be involved in the research more fully? We accept and work with "clients" after they stop being clients. But are people in recovery different from those who remain clients? New ideas need to be tested, and additional models of collaboration need to be tried and evaluated.

There is much to do, much more at stake, and very little time.

REFERENCES

Horowitz, L. (1997). *Emerging Viruses: AIDS, Ebola: Nature, Accident, or Intentional*. Rockport, MA: Tetrahedron.

Morse, S. (Ed.) (1993). *Emerging Viruses*. New York: Oxford University Press.

Index

Page numbers followed by the letter "b" indicate boxed material; those followed by the letter "f" indicate figures; those followed by the letter "n" indicate notes; and those followed by the letter "t" indicate tables.